Kindly Donated

by

Dr Supramaniam

A Colour Atlas of
Respiratory Diseases

D. Geraint James
MA, MD(Cantab.), FRCP(London)

Senior Physician and Dean, Royal Northern Hospital, London
Consultant Physician, Medical Ophthalmology Unit,
St Thomas' Hospital, London
Consulting Physician, Royal Navy
Adjunct Professor, Departments of Medicine and of Epidemiology,
University of Miami School of Medicine, Miama, Florida

Peter R. Studdy
MD, MRCP(UK), FDS, RCS(Eng.)

Consultant Physician,
Cardio Respiratory Unit,
Harefield Hospital, Middlesex

Wolfe Medical Publications Ltd

Copyright © D. G. James, P. R. Studdy, 1981
Published by Wolfe Medical Publications Ltd, 1981
Printed by Royal Smeets Offset b.v.,
Weert, Netherlands
2nd impression 1985
ISBN 0 7234 0762 2

This book is one of the titles in the series of
Wolfe Medical Atlases, a series which brings
together probably the world's largest systematic
published collection of diagnostic colour
photographs.
For a full list of Atlases in the series, plus
forthcoming titles and details of our surgical,
dental and veterinary Atlases, please write to
Wolfe Medical Publications Ltd, Wolfe House,
3 Conway Street, London W1P 6HE.

General Editor, Wolfe Medical Atlases:
G. Barry Carruthers, MD(London)

Contents

(continued)

Preface

This book is designed to complement the bedside studies of medical students, postgraduates working for higher degrees, nurses, and the most helpful growing army of paramedical personnel who are shouldering an increasing and responsible role in the care of patients around the world. Whichever he or she may be, the diagnostician must obtain an adequate history of the disorder and relate it to the abnormal physical signs noted on examination. The next steps in the clinical examination are to link these symptoms and signs with the chest radiograph.

Abnormalities encountered in the chest xray are described in Chapters 1 to 13. Each chapter has a brief, comprehensive description of all abnormalities that may be encountered together with radiographic examples. The student will never regret mastering these abnormal radiographic patterns, because they keep recurring throughout the working life of the doctor and radiologist. However, being a bedside radiologist is not enough. He must integrate the clinical and radiographic abnormalities into a pattern of disease. Thus the chest xray abnormality becomes transformed into the sick patient who may need further investigations before he can be treated accurately. Chapters 14 to 25 correlate these patterns of respiratory disease with the histology or other definitive abnormalities. The respiratory component is often just an incident in a wider multisystem pattern of disease. We have tried to illustrate these multisystem patterns.

This book is a visual representation of Respiratory Diseases. It will be a pictorial supplement to the numerous textbooks on the subject.

Acknowledgements

We gratefully acknowledge the generosity of friends and colleagues who have allowed us to reproduce slides from their collections or helped us in many other ways.

Dr B. Afzelius

Dr D. J. Atherton

Dr Judy Ball

Dr Francoise Basset

Mr M. Bates

Mr T. E. Bucknall

Dr M. Caplin

Dr L. Capel

Dr L. S. Carstairs

Dr P. D. B. Davies

Dr R. J. Davies

Dr Roy Davies

Dr R. Dick

Dr Jennifer Dyson

Dr H. E. Einstein

Dr A. M. Emmerson

Dr D. J. Evans

Mr A. I. Friedmann

Dr I. Kelsey Fry

Dr C. N. Gamble

Dr I. Gordon

Dr C. Hardy

Dr P. Haslam

Dr C. W. Havard

Dr C. J. Heather

Miss Susan Hunt

Dr I. M. James

Dr W. Jones Williams

Dr R. G. Levitt

Professor T. Marshall

Professor E. Florence McKeown

Mr M. McKinnon

Dr J. B. Mitchell

Dr A. Newman-Taylor

Dr L. A. Phillips

The Editor of 'Radiology'

Dr F. C. Rodgers

Dr F. Clifford Rose

Dr A. Sakula

Dr A. M. Salzberg

Mr M.Sanders

Mr R. Sandon

Professor P. Scheuer

Dr R. Seal

Dr O. P. Sharma

Professor Dame Sheila Sherlock

Dr L. E. Siltzbach

Dr G. Sinha

Dr S. Steel

Dr P. Stradling

Miss B. E. Stryjak

Dr A. G. Taylor

Dr A. Tookman

Dr F. R. Vicary

Wellcome Museum of Medical Science

Dr R. A. Womersley

1 Anatomy of the lung

1 Cast of bronchial tree and alveoli. The lungs' primary function is to exchange gas between circulating blood and alveolar air. To perform this function the normal adult lung possesses at least 300 million thin walled distensible air sacs – the alveoli. The alveolar surface area available for gas exchange in the average adult male is estimated at 70 to 85 square metres. At birth the immature lung possesses 20 million alveoli; growth is rapid and the adult number of alveoli is reached at about eight years of age.

The lung-gas exchanging ability can be assessed by measuring the arterial oxygen (PaO_2) and carbon dioxide ($PaCO_2$) tensions. Successful gas exchange depends not only upon normal airways and pulmonary vasculature but also upon intact neuromuscular and cardiac function.

Some naturally circulating substances are metabolised as they pass through the pulmonary capillary bed. Bradykinin, 5-hydroxytryptamine and some prostaglandins are inactivated while angiotensin I is converted to the pressor substance angiotensin II. Some drugs are also metabolised.

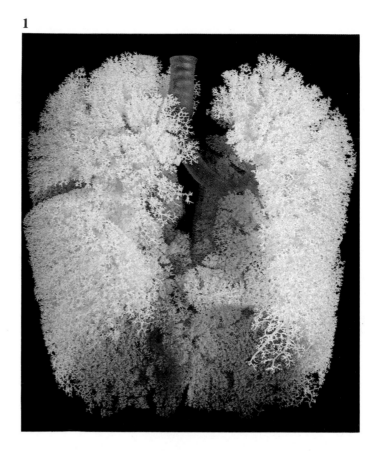

2 Normal adult lung. Histological appearance after pressure fixation with formal saline.

The larger air spaces are alveolar ducts with intact alveoli opening into them.

The normal alveolus is lined by a layer of attenuated epithelial tissue continuous with the lining epithelium of the alveolar ducts and bronchioles.

Two types of alveolar epithelial cells (pneumatocytes) are described; the flattened, plate-like surface, lining alveolar epithelial cells (type 1 pneumatocytes) and the rounded, granular, alveolar epithelial cells (type 2 pneumatocytes), that may produce surfactant.

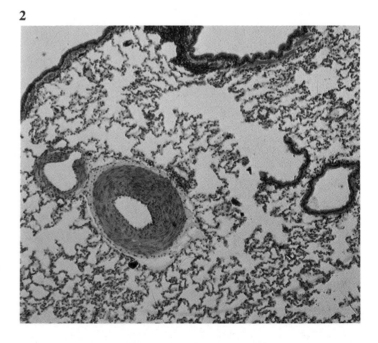

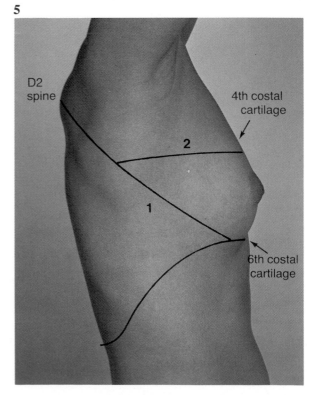

3, 4 and 5 External anatomy. The markings relate to the major fissures. The oblique fissure lies beneath a line joining the second thoracic spine posteriorly to the 6th costochondral junction anteriorly. (Line 1)

The right horizontal fissure follows the 4th intercostal space anteriorly to meet the oblique fissure at the 5th rib in the mid-axillary line. (Line 2)

The position of the nipple varies considerably in the female, but in the male usually lies in the 4th intercostal space.

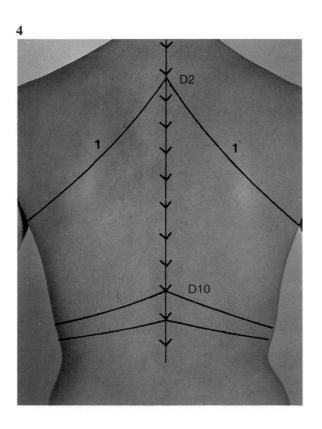

Radiology

6 Posteroanterior view of thorax.
Arrows indicate:
2nd costal cartilage
4th costal cartilage
6th rib in mid clavicular line

1 Trachea

2 First rib

3 Clavicles

4 Superior vena cava

5 Right atrium

6 Right ventricle

7 Left ventricle

8 Left atrium (auricular appendage)

9 Pulmonary artery

10 Inferior vena cava

11 Left cardiophrenic angle

12 Left costophrenic angle

13 Gas in fundus of stomach

14 Pulmonary veins

7 Lateral view of thorax:

1 Trachea

2 Left main bronchus

3 Right main bronchus

4 Ascending thoracic aorta

5 Aortic arch

6 Descending thoracic aorta

7 Right ventricle

8 Left atrium

9 Left ventricle

10 Horizontal fissure

11 Oblique fissure

12 Scapula

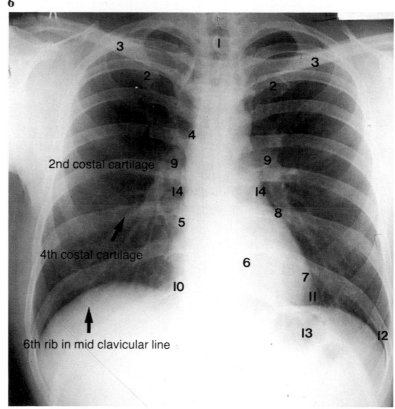

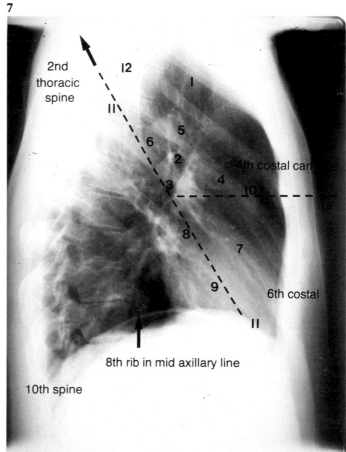

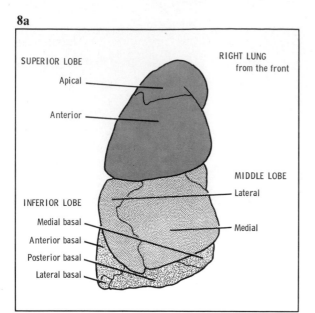

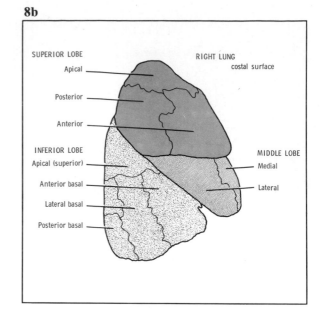

8 Bronchopulmonary segments of the right and left lung.

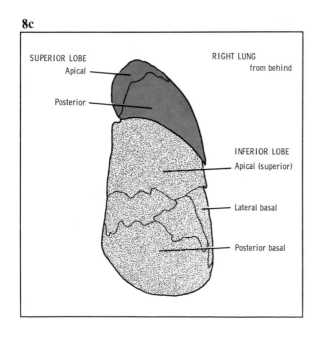

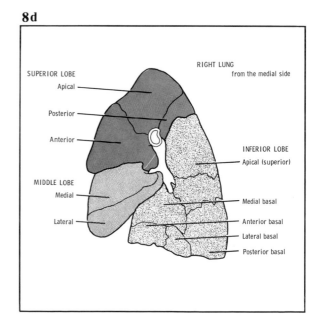

8e

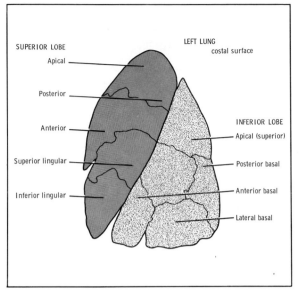

SUPERIOR LOBE

LEFT LUNG
costal surface

Apical

Posterior

Anterior

INFERIOR LOBE

Superior lingular

Apical (superior)

Posterior basal

Inferior lingular

Anterior basal

Lateral basal

8f

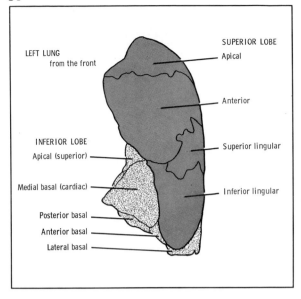

LEFT LUNG
from the front

SUPERIOR LOBE

Apical

Anterior

INFERIOR LOBE

Apical (superior)

Superior lingular

Medial basal (cardiac)

Inferior lingular

Posterior basal

Anterior basal

Lateral basal

8g

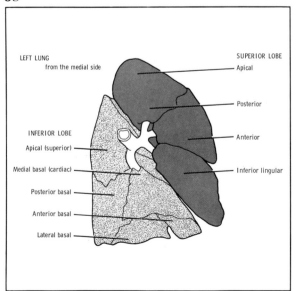

LEFT LUNG
from the medial side

SUPERIOR LOBE

Apical

Posterior

INFERIOR LOBE

Anterior

Apical (superior)

Medial basal (cardiac)

Posterior basal

Inferior lingular

Anterior basal

Lateral basal

8h

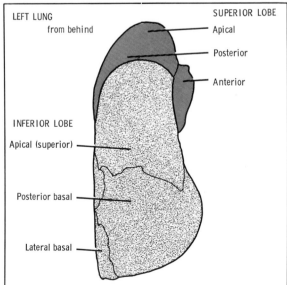

LEFT LUNG
from behind

SUPERIOR LOBE

Apical

Posterior

Anterior

INFERIOR LOBE

Apical (superior)

Posterior basal

Lateral basal

9

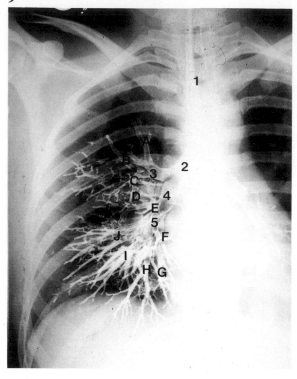

10

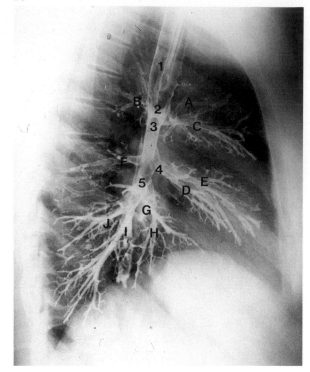

9 Posteroanterior bronchogram of right lung. The right lung is divided into three lobes, the upper, middle and lower, which are further subdivided into broncho-pulmonary segments.

1 Trachea

2 Right main bronchus

3 Right upper lobe bronchus dividing into
  (A) apical segment
  (B) posterior segment
  (C) anterior segment

4 Middle lobe bronchus dividing into
  (D) lateral segment
  (E) medial segment

5 Right lower lobe bronchus
  (F) apical segment
  (G) medial basal segment
  (H) anterior basal segment
  (I) posterior basal segment
  (J) lateral basal segment

10 Lateral bronchogram of right lung.

1 Trachea

2 Right main bronchus

3 Right upper lobe bronchus dividing into
  (A) apical segment
  (B) posterior segment
  (C) anterior segment

4 Middle lobe bronchus dividing into
  (D) lateral segment
  (E) medial segment

5 Right lower lobe bronchus
  (F) apical segment of lower lobe
  (G) medial basal segment
  (H) anterior basal segment
  (I) lateral basal segment
  (J) posterior basal segment

11

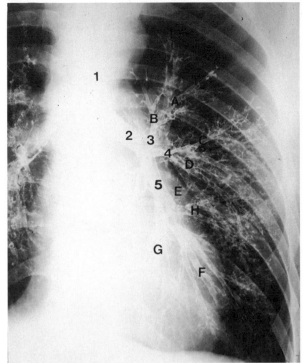

12

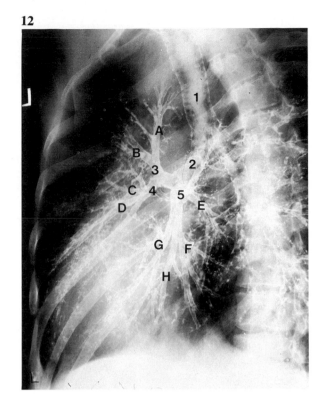

11 Posteroanterior bronchogram of left lung. The left lung is divided into two major lobes by the oblique fissure. The upper lobe and lingula lie above the fissure; the lower lobe lies below.

1 Trachea

2 Left main bronchus

3 Left upper lobe bronchus dividing into
  (A) apico-posterior segment
  (B) anterior segment

4 Lingular lobe bronchus dividing into
  (C) superior segment
  (D) inferior segment

5 Left lower lobe bronchus
  (E) apical segment
  (F) posterior basal segment
  (G) anterior basal segment
  (H) lateral basal segment

12 Lateral bronchogram of left lung. Lateral oblique bronchogram of left lung.

1 Trachea

2 Left main bronchus

3 Left upper lobe bronchus dividing into
  (A) apico-posterior segment
  (B) anterior segment

4 Lingular lobe bronchus dividing into
  (C) superior segment
  (D) inferior segment

5 Left lower lobe bronchus dividing into
  (E) apical segment
  (F) posterior basal segment
  (G) anterior basal segment
  (H) lateral basal segment

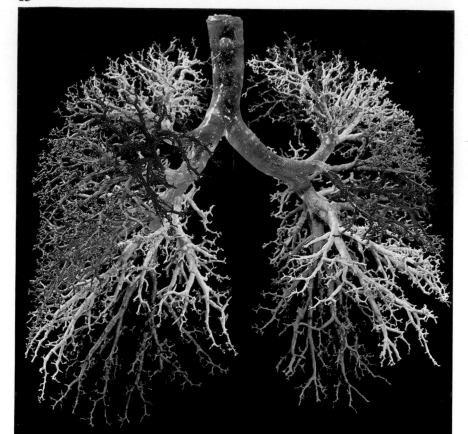

13, 14 and 15 Casts of bronchial tree showing the different bronchopulmonary segments as outlined in the preceding bronchograms.

Lobar bronchi arise from the right or left main bronchi and divide repeatedly into smaller bronchi; after about 10 divisions they give off bronchioles which in turn divide about five times before the terminal bronchioles are reached. The terminal bronchioles are characterised by an absence of supporting cartilage.

The terminal bronchioles then split into respiratory bronchioles and these finally divide into the alveolar ducts, sacs and alveoli.

14

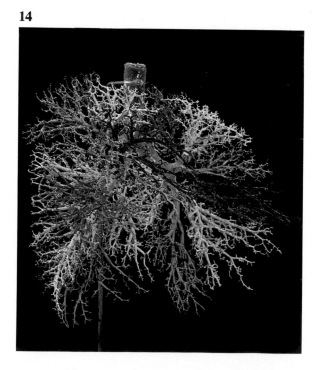

15

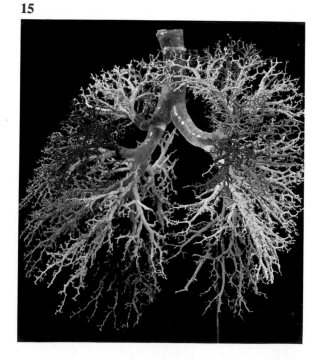

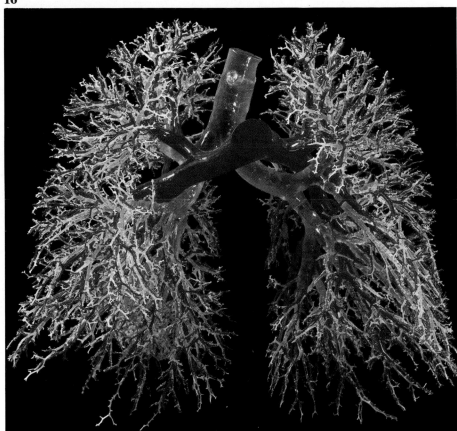

16 Cast of bronchial tree and pulmonary artery. The right and left pulmonary arteries divide in the same manner as the bronchi which they accompany down to the level of the terminal or respiratory bronchioles.

The terminal ramifications of the pulmonary artery do not follow each alveolar duct directly, but drain into the distensible alveolar wall capillary network and then on to the pulmonary veins.

17

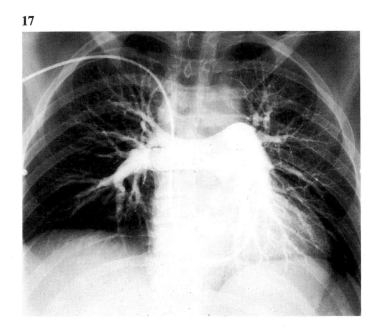

17 Pulmonary angiogram, arterial phase demonstrating the main divisions of the pulmonary artery.

Radioisotope lung imaging

Valuable information, which may show local abnormalities of perfusion or ventilation, can be obtained by radioisotope lung scanning.

18

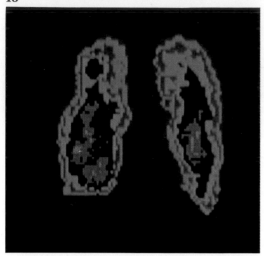

19

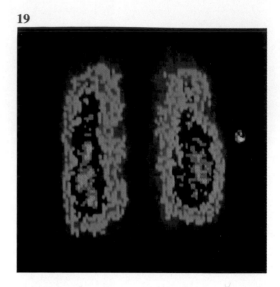

18 and 19 Normal regional perfusion scan of the lung. (**18** anterior view, **19** posterior view.)

Technetium–99m (99TCm) labelled albumin microspheres are injected intravenously. The particles range in size between 15 and 70 μm and impact in the pulmonary circulation.

The distribution of gamma ray emission from the 99TCm labelling is proportional to regional perfusion.

A normal perfusion scan provides firm evidence against a diagnosis of pulmonary embolism.

20

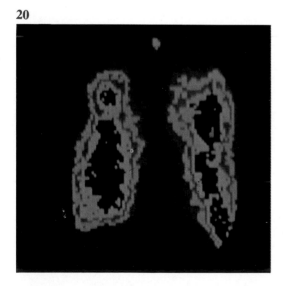

21

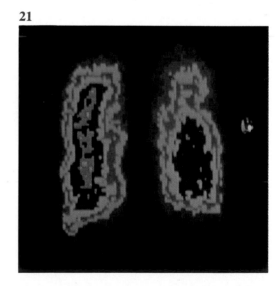

20 and 21 Normal regional ventilation scan of the lung. (**20** anterior view, **21** posterior view.)

Krypton–81m has a half-life of 13 seconds and gives emissions suitable for high resolution gamma camera images.

The gamma emission from any part of the lung after

Krypton inhalation relates to the regional ventilation and provides supplementary information to link with the perfusion scan.

In normal lungs ventilation and perfusion are well matched.

Shape and symmetry of the chest

The external shape of the chest varies widely with body build but some appearances are characteristic.

22

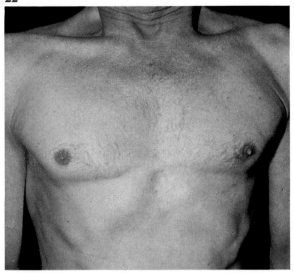

23

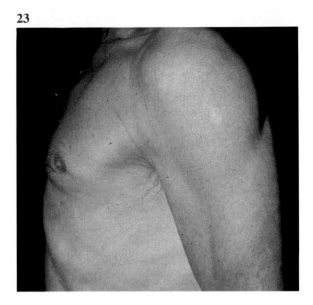

22 and 23 Barrel-shaped chest with increase in antero-posterior diameter is frequently caused by hyperinflation and is seen with emphysema or asthma.

24

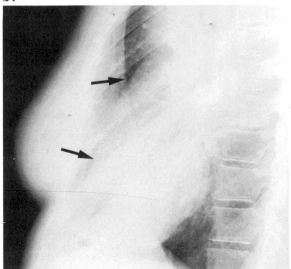

25

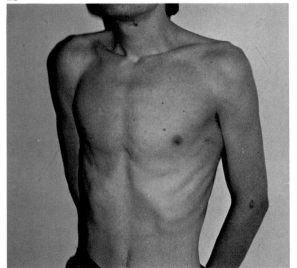

24 Funnel-shaped chest (pectus excavatum) is caused by depression of the lower end of the sternum narrowing the anteroposterior diameter and is a congenital abnormality of no significance. The heart may be displaced to the left. The lateral xray shows the position of the depressed sternum (arrows).

25 Pigeon chest caused by prominence of the upper sternum may follow severe persistent overinflation from childhood asthma.

26

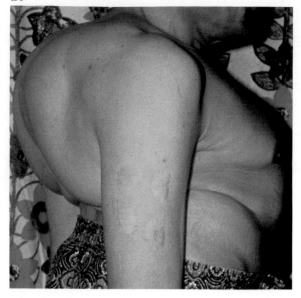

26 **Severe kyphoscoliosis.** There is an increased anterior convexity, exaggerated lumbar lordosis, and moderate lateral deviation producing a secondary rotation of the rib cage. Causes include spinal tuberculosis or infection, trauma, poliomyelitis or congenital spinal abnormalities. In most cases the aetiology is uncertain.

27

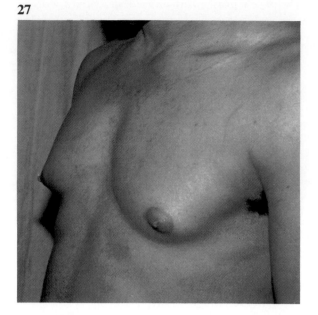

27 **Gynaecomastia.** The male breast may be feminised by oestrogen or oestrogen-like substances. Endogenous oestrogen from tumours or secreted at puberty may be responsible as may exogenous oestrogen or drugs with an oestrogen-like structure such as digitalis, spironolactone and the phenothiazines.

28

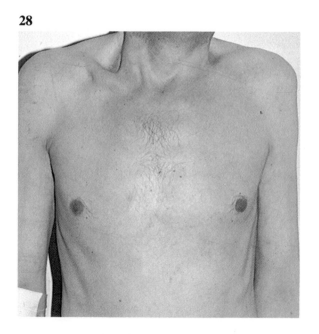

28 **Flattening of upper anterior chest** as a consequence of fibrosis of the underlying lung. The position of the trachea and mediastinum is deviated towards the fibrotic lung.

29

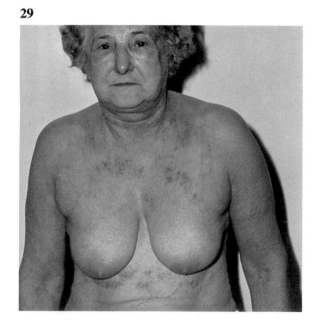

29 **Superior vena caval obstruction.** The distended veins over the lower chest, non-pulsatile distension of the jugular veins, swollen arms and bloated face are characteristic.

2 Pleural effusion

In health there is a thin layer of fluid in the pleural space. Excess fluid may accumulate by transudation or exudation in a wide variety of conditions. A small effusion may be undetectable but if 500 ml or more of fluid are present chest-wall movement is diminished, percussion note breath sounds and vocal resonance reduced and vocal fremitus absent.

Breathlessness is a common clinical feature with large effusions and pleurisy a common feature of pleural inflammation.

The effusion may be:

(a) Massive with mediastinal shift.
(b) Moderate in size. Whatever the aetiology, pleural fluid often presents the familiar radiographic appearance of a homogeneous opacity with a concave upper border higher laterally than medially, the so-called pleural meniscus. Actually there is nothing in the pleural sac of this shape. If it were possible to solidify the fluid, the lung would be found encased in a cup-shaped cast, thick at the base and tapering to a fine edge at the top. The meniscus is a tangential radiographic projection of the lateral side of this cast.
(c) Minimal. The costophrenic angle may either be obliterated, or may only be visible posteriorly in the lateral film. A lateral decubitus film may help to distinguish free fluid from thickened pleura.
(d) Loculated. This may be interlobar, parietal, perilobar or subperilobar or subpulmonary.

The fluid may be blood, lymph, pus, transudate (protein content <30 g/litre) or an exudate (protein content >30 g/litre). The nature of the fluid can only be determined by visual and laboratory inspection of an aspirated specimen which should be obtained in all cases of pleural effusion except those obviously cardiac in origin.

Cytological examination is essential. The presence of malignant cells in disseminated cancer is diagnostic. Polymorphs suggest an effusion secondary to bacterial infection while lymphocytes are found in chronic serous effusions or tuberculosis. Eosinophils may be seen in effusions complicating allergic lung disease, polyarteritis nodosa, or after minor haemorrhage into the pleural space such as may accompany pulmonary infarction.

Bacterial examination by direct smear and culture for aerobic and anaerobic bacteria, fungi, and mycobacteria should be routine when infection is suspected. However, pleural biopsy is more likely to be diagnostic than culture in serous tuberculous effusions.

Biochemical analysis may be diagnostic when high amylase concentrations are found in pancreatitis.

Estimating the fluid protein content is seldom of important diagnostic help. On the rare occasions when there is clinical doubt about the nature of a serous effusion, the protein content usually is in the borderline range of 30 g/litre and does not discriminate between an exudate or transudate.

Transudate is usually caused by congestive cardiac failure; most commonly right-sided, frequently bilateral. Less common causes are hepatic and renal failure, Meig's syndrome of ovarian fibroma with right pleural transudate, anaemia, and superior vena caval obstruction caused by cancer and Behçet's syndrome.

Exudates are most often caused by infections, particularly tuberculosis and malignancy. Neoplastic effusions are usually caused by bronchial carcinoma and less often by alveolar cell carcinoma, metastases, mesothelioma, lymphoma or multiple myeloma. Exudates may also be a feature of rheumatoid arthritis, systemic lupus, pulmonary infarction, subphrenic abscess, and chronic idiopathic lymphoedema (yellow-nail syndrome).

Haemothorax is caused by trauma, surgery, pulmonary infarction, rupture of an aneurysm or adhesions from a spontaneous pneumothorax, anticoagulant therapy or a coagulation disorder.

Chylothorax is caused by trauma, thoracic surgery, or mediastinal malignancy. The condition is rarely spontaneous.

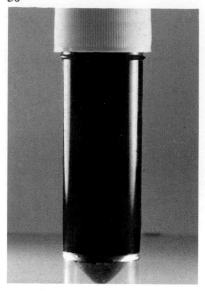

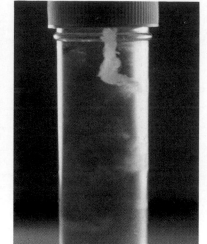

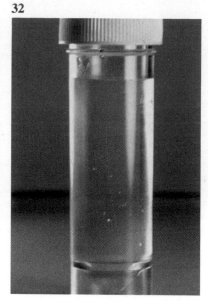

30 Appearances of pleural effusion. Blood-stained pleural effusion commonly occurs with pulmonary infarction or malignancy. Rarely are tuberculous effusions heavily blood-stained.

31 Yellow exudate pleural effusion. The exudates have a high protein content (>30 g/litre) and a high specific gravity (>1.015). The appearance is similar to plasma and is caused by the high protein content which may clot. Turbid fluid results from a high cell count.

32 Clear transudated pleural effusions. Transudates have a low protein content (<30 g/litre) and a low specific gravity (<1.015).

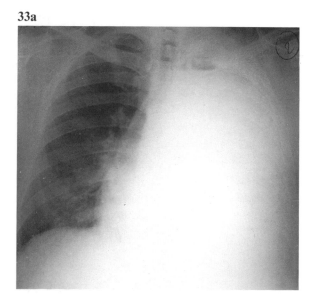

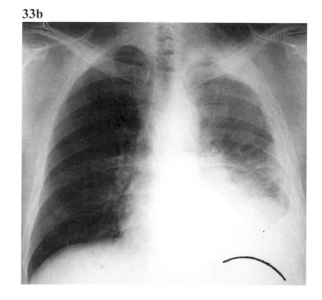

33a Massive malignant pleural effusion. The mediastinum is deviated to the right and the diaphragm depressed by the weight of fluid. Tuberculosis or haemothorax may result in similar massive effusions.

33b Massive malignant pleural effusions. Five litres of fluid were aspirated with considerable relief of symptoms. The upper border of the fluid appears concave. Note the central position of the mediastinum.

34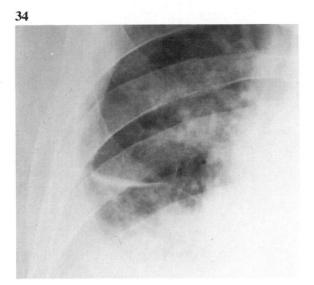

35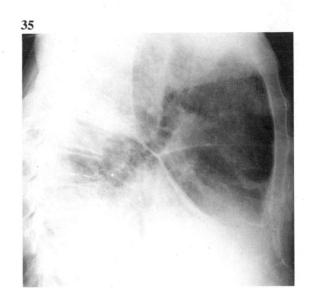

34 and 35   Moderate right pleural effusion. The lateral view shows the presence of fluid in the major fissure. The fluid density results in a diffuse opacity over the lower thoracic vertebrae.

36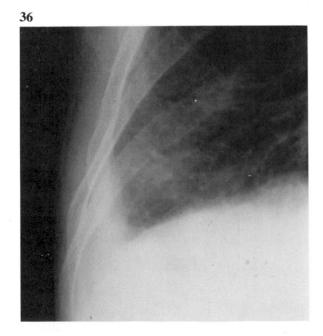

37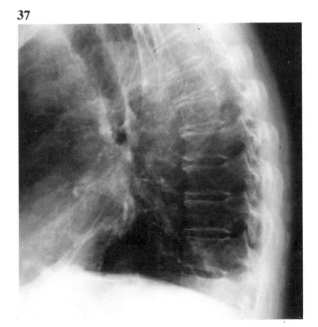

36 and 37   Small pleural effusion caused by left ventricular failure. The costophrenic angle is blunted by fluid which the lateral film shows to lie posteriorly.

38

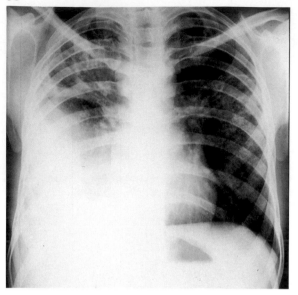

39

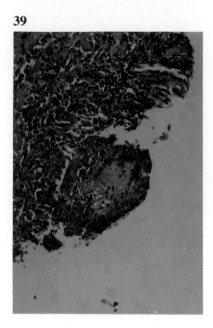

38 Post-primary tuberculosis in an immigrant. The bilateral bronchopneumonic shadowing is caused by tuberculous pneumonia. The diagnosis was established by pleural biopsy which shows caseating granulomas; no acid-fast bacilli were found in the pleural fluid.

39 Caseating granulomas in pleural biopsy tissue confirmed the diagnosis of tuberculosis.

40

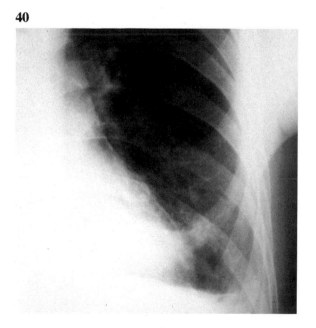

41

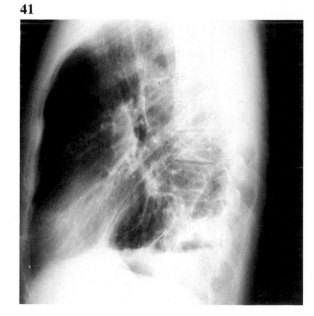

40 and 41 Pulmonary embolus. A moderate-sized haemorrhagic effusion developed soon after infarction of the left lung.

42 **Right pleural transudate** caused by high-output cardiac failure in a patient with Paget's disease. The very dense enlarged right clavicle is the clue to the diagnosis. The characteristic feature of Paget's disease is the increased resorption of bone accompanied by some increase in bone formation.

When resorption predominates the bones are brittle, soft and very vascular. This latter feature accounts for the increased warmth noted over affected bones. In widespread disease the increased blood flow through the skeleton may result in high-output cardiac failure. This patient's disease involved the femur, pelvis and lumbosacral spine in addition to the right clavicle.

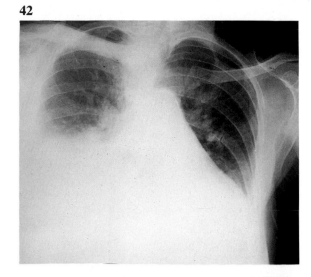

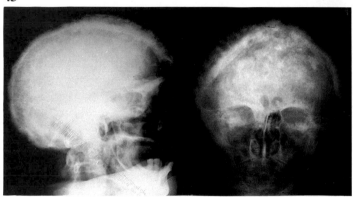

43 **Paget's disease.** The outer table of the cranium is thickened with irregular increases in bone density. The skull xray shows a characteristic fluffy or cotton-wool appearance.

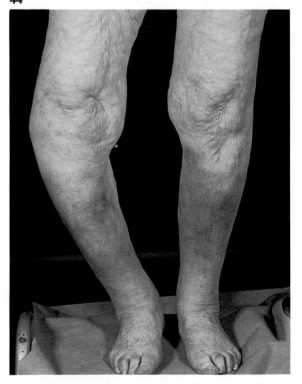

44 **Paget's disease.** Deformity with bowing of the right leg. The long bones are often deformed in this way and thickening of the cortex is usually seen on the convex side of the curve.

The disease is frequently asymmetrical and patchy in distribution. The femur and pelvic bones are most commonly involved followed by the skull, tibia, lumbosacral spine, dorsal spine, ribs and clavicles in that order.

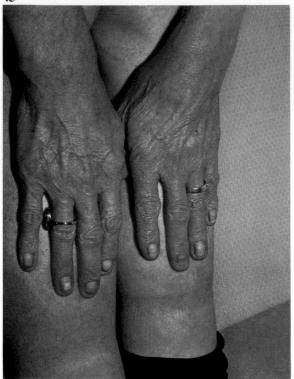

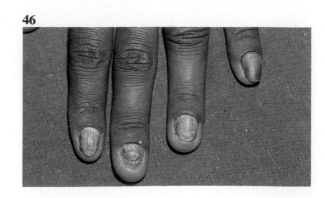

46 Yellow-nail syndrome. Growth of the green-yellow nails is reduced and occasionally a nail may be shed.

45 Yellow-nail syndrome. Pleural effusions may rarely be associated with primary lymphoedema of the legs and yellow discolouration of the nails. The common link to these three features may be a developmental deficiency of the lymphatics.

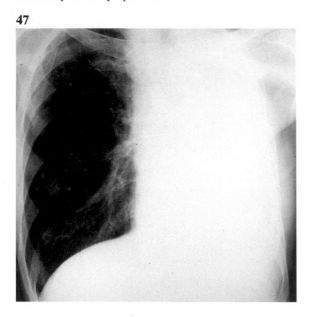

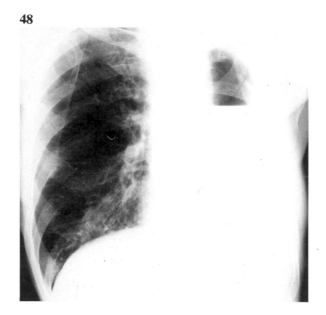

47 Post-pneumonectomy pleural effusion. The pleural cavity normally fills with fluid after pneumonectomy. The mediastinum and heart are deviated to the left, the operated side.

48 Bronchopleural fistula. The xray was taken after the patient had expectorated 3 litres of straw-coloured fluid. The fluid level indicates that air has entered the chest cavity. The bronchial stump may be eroded by infection or, as in this case, by recurrent malignancy eight months after pneumonectomy.

3 Pneumothorax and mediastinal emphysema

A pneumothorax develops when air escapes into the pleural cavity allowing the underlying lung to collapse.

Four different types of pneumothorax are described:

1 Primary spontaneous pneumothorax. Some 85 per cent of cases occur in males, most commonly between 20 and 40 years of age and of ectomorphic physique. The recurrence rate is 20 per cent after the first episode and 50 per cent if two episodes of pneumothorax have occurred.

Primary spontaneous pneumothorax is usually caused by rupture of small subpleural bullae 1 cm to 2 cm in diameter at the lung apex. It is also a common complication of histiocytosis and connective tissue disorders such as Marfan's syndrome.

2 Secondary pneumothorax is common in chronic bronchitis and emphysema caused by rupture of subpleural bullae and may complicate pneumonia, lung abscess, tuberculosis, asthma, cystic fibrosis or bronchial carcinoma.

3 Traumatic pneumothorax from penetrating injuries of the chest wall.

4 Artificial or induced pneumothorax.

The mechanical problems caused by a pneumothorax may be considered as:

a) Closed pneumothorax. The hole in the visceral pleura closes spontaneously. Irrespective of the cause, a pneumothorax slowly decreases in size when the air leak seals. If the lung and pleura are healthy, a 50 per cent pneumothorax takes about 40 days to be fully reabsorbed.

b) Open pneumothorax. Air leaks through the visceral pleura preventing re-expansion of the lung.

c) Tension pneumothorax. A valvular mechanism at the site of pleural air leak allows a progressive increase in intrapleural pressure which compresses the affected lung and the mediastinal structures against the contralateral lung. This is potentially a fatal condition.

49

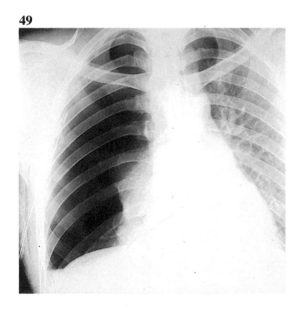

49 Spontaneous pneumothorax presenting with pleuritic pain and mild dyspnoea. A young fit patient may tolerate a large pneumothorax, whereas a small pneumothorax in an elderly bronchitic may cause life-threatening respiratory failure.

50

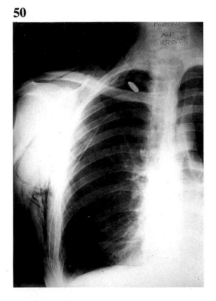

50 Spontaneous pneumothorax with complete collapse of the right lung and shift of the mediastinum. An intercostal tube was inserted to re-expand the lung. Air has immediately tracked outside the drainage tube, producing surgical emphysema in the soft tissues of the chest wall and neck. A characteristic 'crackling' sensation can be elicited on palpation.

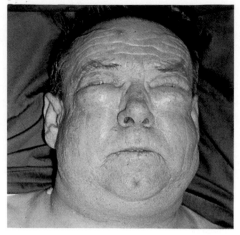

51 Surgical emphysema of the face. Gross surgical emphysema of the chest wall, neck and face as a consequence of air leaking through an open pneumothorax.

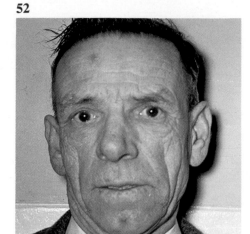

52 Surgical emphysema. The same patient appears normal two weeks later.

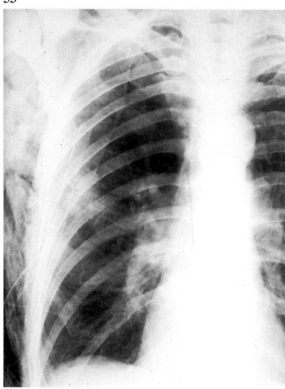

53 Surgical emphysema of the chest wall. Air outlines the pectoral muscles.

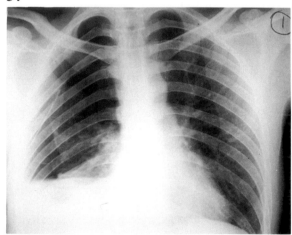

54 Right haemopneumothorax. This occurred when a second drainage tube was inserted. The rib spaces are narrowed as a result of the collapse of the underlying lung.

55

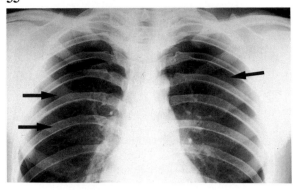

55 Bilateral spontaneous pneumothorax. This young man with Marfan's syndrome had bilateral apical bullae and presented with bilateral pneumothoraces (arrows). A right pleurectomy was performed and the left side was treated by talc pleurodesis.

56

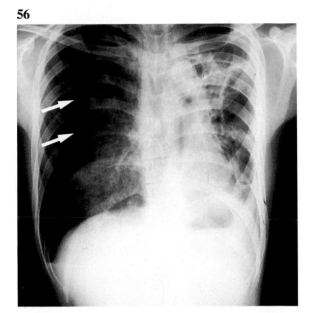

56 Secondary right pneumothorax in a patient with a destroyed left lung. This is a potentially life-threatening situation and early pleurodesis or pleurectomy may prevent a fatal recurrence. This patient had extensive fibrosis from healed pulmonary tuberculosis.

57

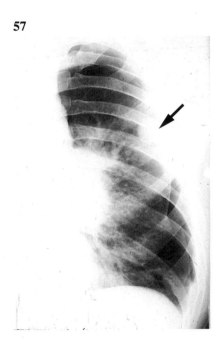

57 Traumatic left pneumothorax after needle biopsy of a peripheral lesion. An enlarged hilum caused by oat-cell carcinoma is also visible. Small pneumothoraces commonly occur after aspiration needle biopsy but they seldom require drainage.

58

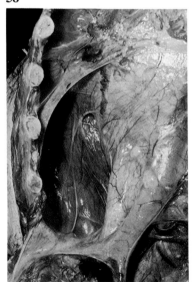

58 Tension pneumothorax. The pleural space is visible in the necropsy specimen.

Mediastinal emphysema

Air may directly enter the mediastinum from a ruptured bronchus or oesophagus or indirectly along the pulmonary vessels after rupture of the alveoli.

59

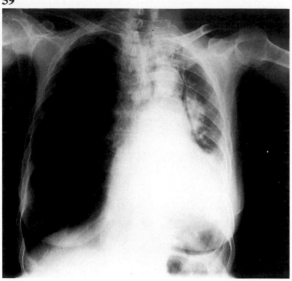

60

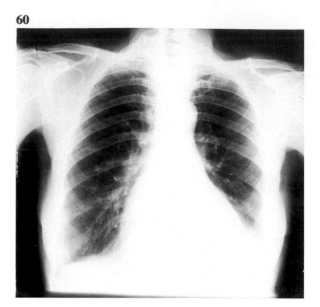

59 Mediastinal emphysema. The left lung is partially collapsed and the trachea deviated to the left. Air in the mediastinum appears as a narrow translucent halo outlining the heart and aortic arch (arrow). The left main bronchus was occluded by a tenacious mucus plug in this asthmatic patient.

60 Mediastinal emphysema. The left lung re-expanded when the mucus plug was aspirated.

4 The diaphragm

The diaphragm is the most important respiratory muscle. In normal quiet breathing it is responsible for three-quarters of the inhaled total volume. The intercostal muscles contribute the remaining one-quarter. Unilateral paralysis reduces the ventilating capacity by some 20 per cent but is well tolerated unless the lungs are diseased. Even total bilateral diaphragmatic paralysis is compatible with life because of partial compensation by other muscles of respiration.

Embryological development is complex; the largest portion originates from the fourth mesodermal somite bringing innervation from C4 with minor contributions from C3 and C5 via the phrenic nerve. Development is completed about the twelfth week of foetal life.

Numerous congenital abnormalities may occur. Failure of fusion allows the gut to lie in the thorax and critically impede development of the bronchial tree, which is only completed at 16 weeks of intrauterine life. Both normal diaphragms have a characteristic humped shape on the xray and are well defined. Flattening usually is caused by hyperinflation and loss of outline indicates adjacent pleural or pulmonary disease.

The diaphragm may be elevated or depressed by disease above or below it; it may be paralysed by phrenic nerve involvement, or it may be the site of congenital or traumatic herniation.

Abnormal position of diaphragm	Possible causes
Unilateral elevation	Phrenic nerve paralysis
	Pulmonary embolism
	Basal and diaphragmatic pleurisy
	Bornholm disease
	Pulmonary resection
	Atelectasis
	Hepatomegaly or splenomegaly
	Subphrenic abscess
	Eventration — Partial right-sided / Complete left-sided
Bilateral elevation	Pregnancy
	Ascites
	Paralytic ileus
Unilateral depression	Pneumothorax
	Basal cyst with air-trapping
Bilateral depression	Emphysema
	Status asthmaticus
	Carcinoma of trachea

61

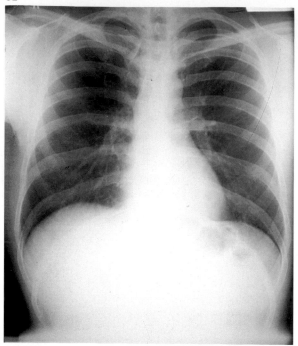

62

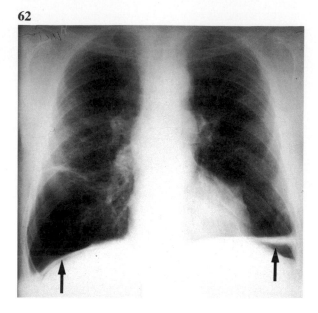

62 Air beneath the diaphragm. The diaphragm only appears distinctive when air is present both above and below it.

61 Normal appearance of the diaphragm. The right hemidiaphragm is normally higher than the left; the common explanation is that the underlying liver elevates the diaphragm. However, studies of isolated dextrocardia show that the position of the diaphragm is most influenced by the mass of the overlying heart.

63

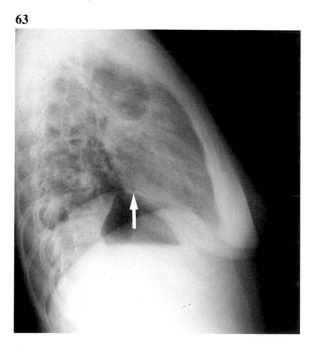

64

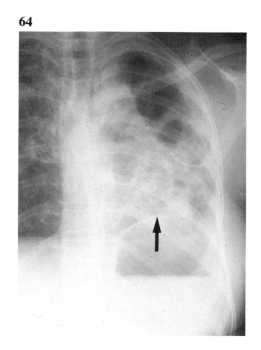

63 and 64 Elevated left diaphragm. The left lung has been destroyed by tuberculosis resulting in loss of volume with shift of the mediastinum and elevation of the diaphragm. The position of the gastric air bubble on the lateral film is unusually high.

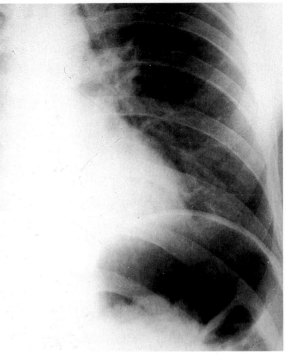

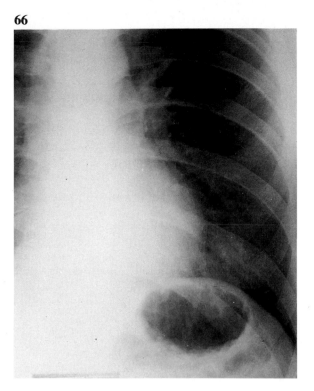

65 Elevated left diaphragm. Considerable gaseous distension of the stomach has elevated the left diaphragm.

66 Elevated left diaphragm. A repeat film shows less gas and a normal position of the diaphragm. (same patient as **65**).

67

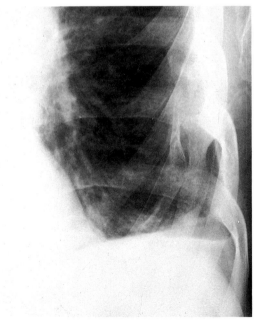

67 Fixed elevated left diaphragm. Drainage of empyema in childhood has left a thickened pleura.

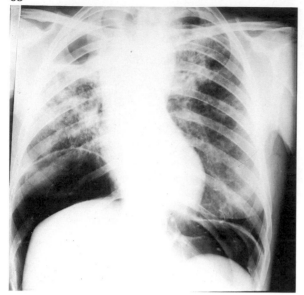

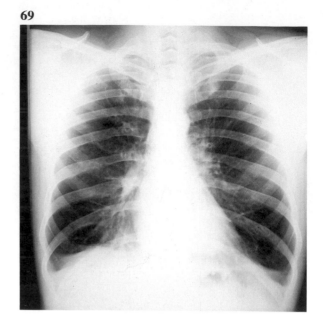

68 Bilateral elevation of diaphragm by therapeutic pneumoperitoneum induced as treatment for active cavitating pulmonary tuberculosis in the preantibiotic era. The very high position of the right diaphragm is in part caused by a right phrenic nerve section.

69 Bilateral descent of diaphragm. Scalloping of the diaphragm occurred during an acute attack of asthma. The costal attachments become visible when hyperinflation depresses the diaphragm muscle.

Diaphragmatic hernia

Congenital or acquired defects of the diaphragm may allow the abdominal contents to herniate into the thorax.

Large congenital hernias are rare but when present cause respiratory embarrassment in infancy.

At least three-quarters of diaphragmatic hernias occur through the oesophageal hiatus, usually are acquired, and present with symptoms from middle-age onwards.

Three main types of oesophageal hiatus hernias are described.

70a Sliding or oesophagogastric hernia. 90 per cent are of this type. The gastric fundus ascends through the functionally incompetent hiatal orifice into the posterior mediastinum. Symptoms are variable and caused by reflux.

70b Rolling or paraoesophageal. The gastric cardia is normally placed but the greater curvature or rarely the whole stomach ascends into the posterior mediastinum. Symptoms are from recurrent gastric volvulus rather than reflux.

70c Mixed hiatus hernia.

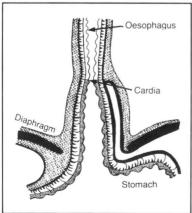

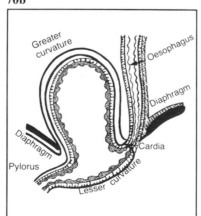

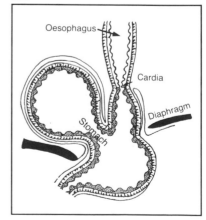

71

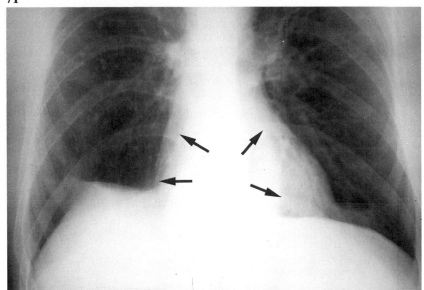

71, 72 and 73 Sliding oesophageal hiatal hernia (oesophagogastric). The portion of stomach lying above the diaphragm is seen as a radiolucency lying behind the heart in the posterior mediastinum (**71** and **72**). Fluid levels may be seen on occasion. The barium-meal investigation (**73**) outlines the portion of stomach lying above the diaphragm in the sliding hernia. More than 90 per cent of all diaphragmatic hernias occur through the oesophageal hiatus. Various types are described.

72

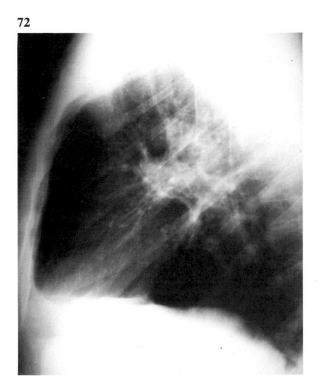

73

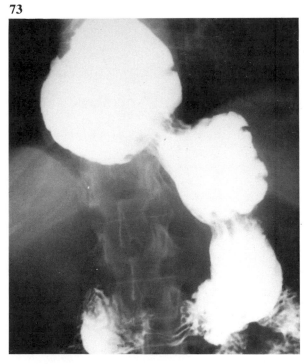

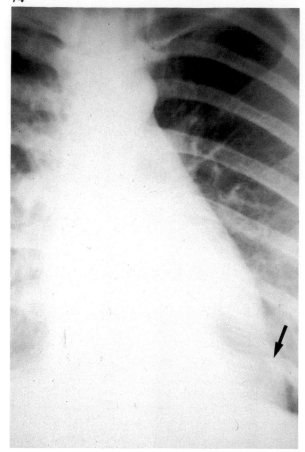

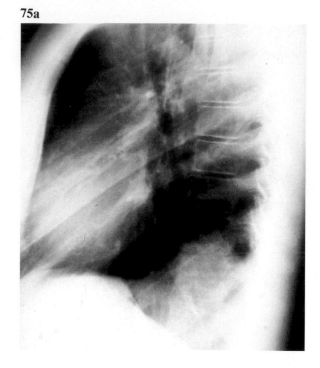

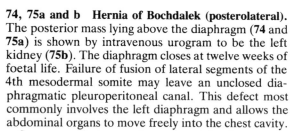

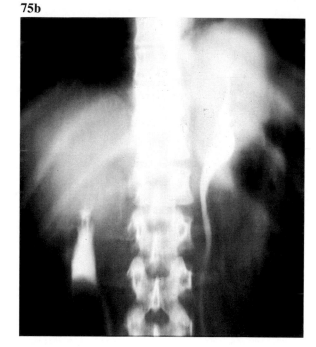

74, 75a and b   Hernia of Bochdalek (posterolateral).
The posterior mass lying above the diaphragm (**74** and
75a) is shown by intravenous urogram to be the left
kidney (**75b**). The diaphragm closes at twelve weeks of
foetal life. Failure of fusion of lateral segments of the
4th mesodermal somite may leave an unclosed diaphragmatic pleuroperitoneal canal. This defect most
commonly involves the left diaphragm and allows the
abdominal organs to move freely into the chest cavity.

Severe respiratory embarrassment in the neonate
may draw attention to the diaphragmatic defect.

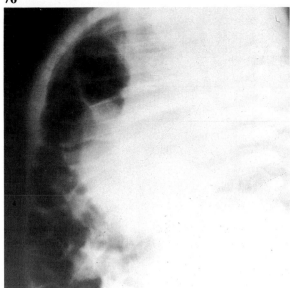

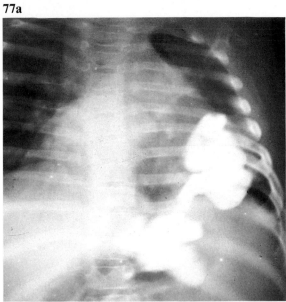

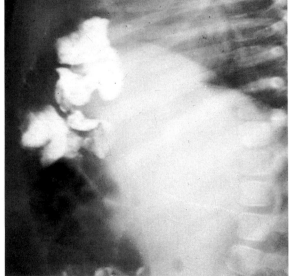

76, 77a and b   Foramen of Morgagni hernia (anterior). The defect lies between the sternal and costal attachments of the diaphragm: it is more common on the right side. These hernias are seldom as extensive as the posterolateral type and rarely cause respiratory embarrassment. Omental fat or intestine may herniate through the foramen. This example shows small bowel containing barium and air-filled large bowel.

76   Lateral view of chest and upper abdomen;

77a   PA after barium meal;

77b   Lateral view of chest and upper abdomen.

5 Hilar adenopathy

The hilar shadows

The normal hilar shadows are composed of the pulmonary arteries and their main branches, the upper lobe pulmonary veins, the major bronchi and the lymph glands. The bronchi contribute little to the hilar shadows, because they are filled with air, and normal lymph nodes are too small to add size or density. It is important to distinguish enlarged vascular shadows from lymphadenopathy; this is usually evident in the lateral film. There are significant differences between the causes of unilateral and bilateral hilar enlargement, so it is important to establish the extent of involvement, if necessary by tomography or even angiography.

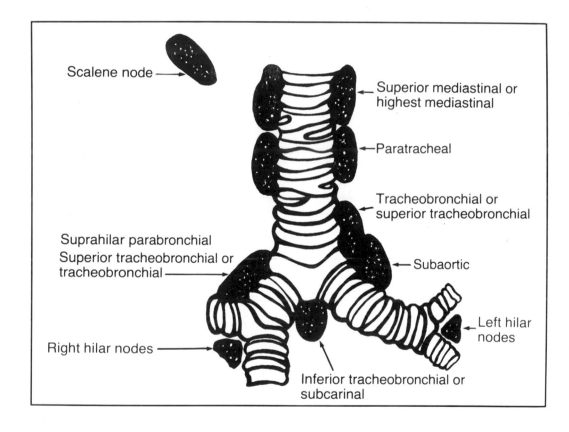

Unilateral hilar lymphadenopathy

Causes	Confirmation
Bronchial carcinoma	Bronchoscopic biopsy Sputum cytology
Tuberculosis	Strongly positive tuberculin test Pulmonary lesion (Ghon focus) Sputum culture
Sarcoidosis Histoplasmosis Coccidioidomycosis	As for bilateral hilar lymphadenopathy

Bilateral hilar lymphadenopathy

Causes	Confirmation
Sarcoidosis	Erythema nodosum Uveitis Fibreoptic bronchoscopy Kveim test Serum angiotensin-converting enzyme
Tuberculosis	Migrant communities Tuberculin skin test conversion Search for mycobacteria
Lymphoma	Ill, febrile, losing weight Fibreoptic bronchoscopy
Metastases	Lymph node biopsy
Coccidioidomycosis Histoplasmosis	Endemic zones Erythema nodosum Skin test Serum antibodies
Beryllium disease	History of exposure Accompanying pulmonary lesions Skin test Normal angiotensin-converting enzyme

78

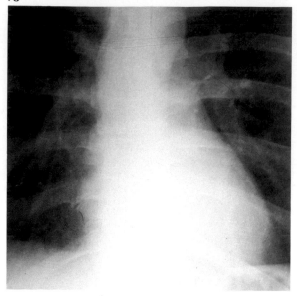

78 Normal hilar shadows are usually of equal density and size, the left hilum being 1 cm to 1.5 cm higher than the right.

79

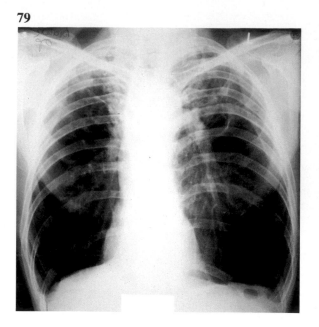

79 Elevated hilar shadows as a consequence of upper lobe shrinkage caused by pulmonary tuberculosis.

80

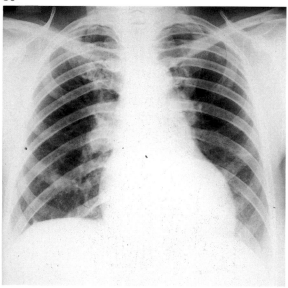

80 Bilateral hilar enlargement caused by cor pulmonale in a patient with long-standing chronic lung disease. There is cardiac enlargement and considerable dilatation of the pulmonary arteries.

81

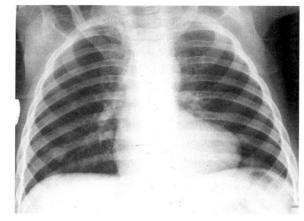

81 Bilateral small hilar shadows commonly occur in cyanotic congenital heart disease, for example tetralogy of Fallot, tricuspid atresia, truncus arteriosus and transposition of the great vessels. (The T's serve as a mnemonic.)

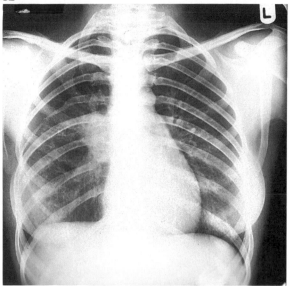

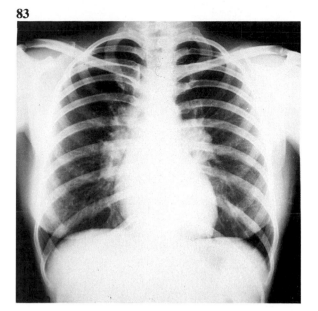

82 Unilateral right hilar gland enlargement. The enlarged right paratracheal gland in this 25-year-old immigrant was caused by tuberculosis. Carcinoma of the bronchus may give a similar appearance.

83 Bilateral hilar gland enlargement in sarcoidosis. There is also pulmonary infiltration. A clear uninvolved zone is visible between the nodes and the central hilum. The hilar and right paratracheal nodes are most commonly involved in sarcoidosis and also in lymphoma.

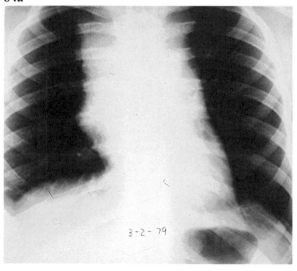

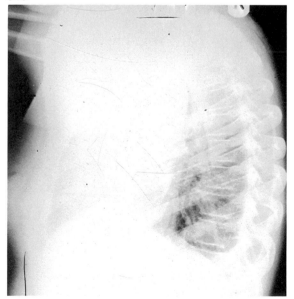

84a and b Anterior mediastinal glandular enlargement in an 11-year-old girl with acute leukaemia. The upper mediastinal shadow is widened and the retrosternal space obliterated by the enlarged glands.

6 Pulmonary nodules and masses

Solitary pulmonary nodule

The solitary circumscribed pulmonary nodule presents a common diagnostic dilemma. Benign lesions seldom warrant surgery whereas early excision of a localised carcinoma may be curative. Calcification is common in benign hamartomas or healed granulomas. Stable uncalcified lesions and calcified nodules in patients less than 35 years of age seldom require surgery and may be observed. In the older patient a solitary nodule is more likely to be malignant so tissue diagnosis is essential. The solitary nodule is spherical or oval, relatively well-defined, less than about 5 cm in diameter, and lies within the lung. The causes and diagnostic measures are listed (Table on page 45).

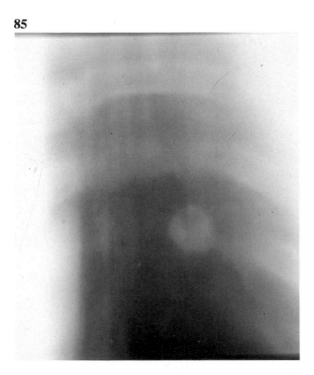

85 Solitary nodule caused by bronchial adenoma. The sharply circumscribed margin occurs in about 25 per cent of bronchial carcinomas and some tuberculomas (tomographic view).

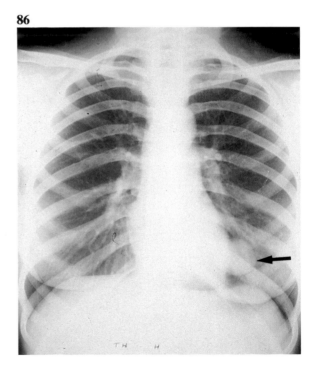

86 Hamartoma is the most common benign pulmonary tumour. Calcification is common (40 per cent).

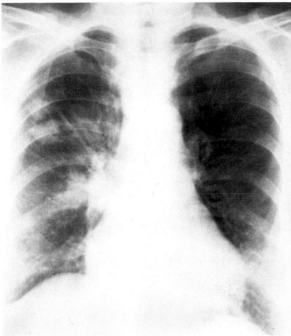

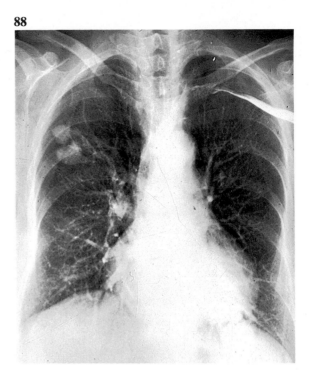

87 Arteriovenous fistula. Often well circumscribed and never calcifies. This vascular abnormality, often multiple, is caused by the persistence of foetal capillary anastomoses between the arterial and venous pulmonary circulation.

88 Pulmonary angiography is diagnostic. Small lesions are asymptomatic. In large lesions a major right-to-left shunt of unoxygenated blood may occur with dyspnoea, cyanosis, polycythaemia and finger clubbing.

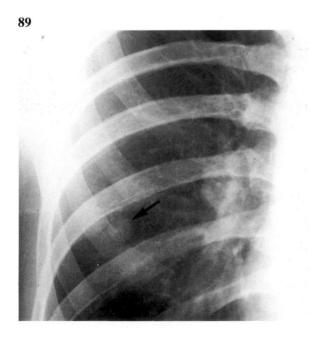

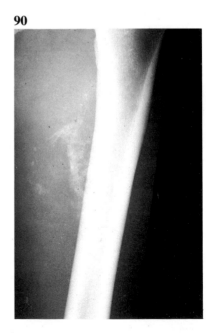

89 Solitary pulmonary metastases from osteosarcoma of femur.

90 Osteosarcoma of femur (same patient as **89**).

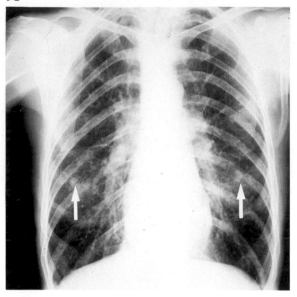

91 Soft tissue shadows may simulate an intra-pulmonary nodule. Nipple shadows are often seen on standard chest radiographs (arrowed).

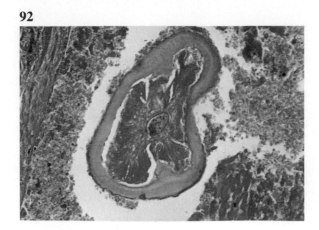

92 Dirofilaria immitis, the dog heart worm, is an unusual cause of a solitary pulmonary nodule. The dead worm impacts in a branch of the pulmonary artery, inciting thrombosis and infarction. The condition is seen in Japan, Australia and the south-eastern USA.

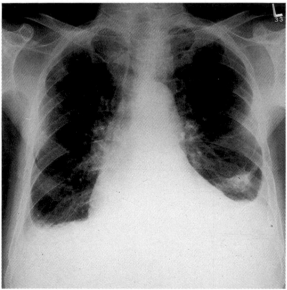

93 Loculated interlobar pleural effusion in the left mid-zone may simulate a nodule on the PA film. The large heart, congested lung fields, bilateral pleural and loculated effusion are caused by right heart failure. The lateral view (not shown) confirmed the presence of fluid in the oblique fissure.

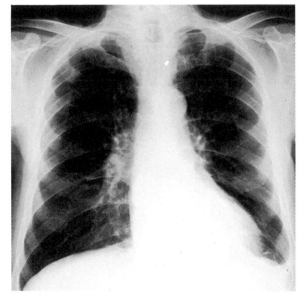

94 Loculated interlobar effusion. (Vanishing tumour.) Improvement as a result of prescribing diuretics. The heart is smaller, lung fields less congested and loculated effusion resolved. Only a small effusion remains at the left costophrenic angle.

Solitary pulmonary nodule

Causes	Confirmation
Bronchial carcinoma	Fibreoptic bronchoscopy
Alveolar cell carcinoma	Aspiration needle biopsy Sputum cytology
Metastasis	Aspiration needle biopsy Search for primary neoplasm
Bronchial adenoma (carcinoid)	Bronchoscopy Aspiration needle biopsy
Granuloma caused by tuberculosis, histoplasmosis or coccidioidomycosis	Endemic zones Calcification in tuberculosis and histoplasmosis but uncommon in coccidioidomycosis Skin tests Serum antibodies
Hydatid cyst (echinococcal)	Endemic zones Lobulated; lower lobe distribution Casoni skin test Complement fixation test Eosinophilia Liver scan for hepatic cysts
Dirofilaria immitis (dog heartworm)	Biopsy reveals eosinophilic granuloma
Arteriovenous aneurysm	Teliangectasia of lips and nasal mucosa Angiography
Hamartoma	Calcification frequent Aspiration biopsy

Pulmonary masses

A large intrathoracic opacity over 5 cm in diameter is usually malignant, and is caused by a bronchial carcinoma, metastases, lymphoma, plasmacytoma or a mesothelioma. Benign tumours include hamartoma, fibroma, leiomyoma, lipoma, neurofibroma and chondroma. Granulomas rarely cause such large lesions but cryptococcoma (torulosis) may occur in the lower lobes, and an aspergilloma (fungus ball or mycetoma) may occupy a chronic lung cavity. Intrapulmonary sequestration may appear to be a fluid-filled cyst in the posterobasal segment of the right lower lobe. Large solitary masses may also be caused by hydatid cyst, encysted interlobar pleural effusion and pulmonary infarcts. (*See* page 262.)

95

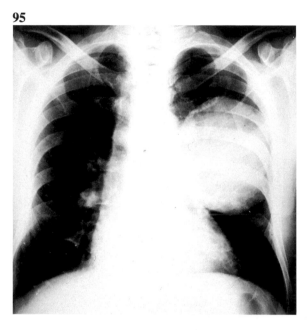

95 Large mass in left upper zone. The patient was asymptomatic and declined any investigation. Post-mortem examination revealed coronary artery disease (the cause of death) and a large fibroma.

96

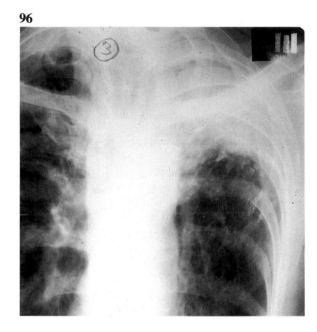

96 Large aspergilloma in old tuberculous cavity. A translucent halo surrounds the fungus ball.

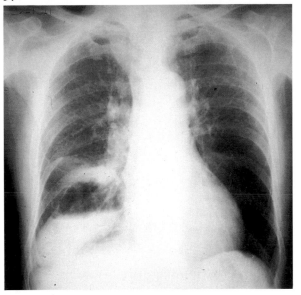

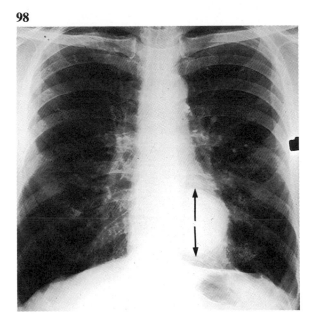

97 Bleeding into a basal cyst simulated a large tumour in the right lower lobe. Aspiration biopsy revealed blood and this repeat film demonstrates a fluid level.

98 Neurilemmoma (neurofibroma). A dense circular retrocardiac opacity. These benign tumours are often clinically silent. Adjacent ribs may be splayed or eroded as size increases.

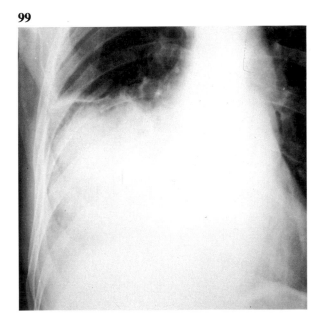

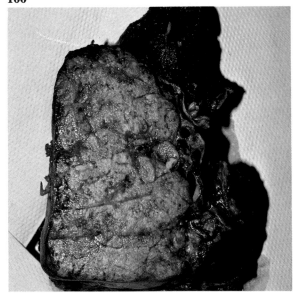

99 and 100 Squamous cell carcinoma infiltrating the right lower lobe. The necropsy specimen of the whole right lung shows tumour invading the lower lobe. A mass of this size is unlikely to be benign, but lipomas or neurogenic tumours may attain a massive size.

101

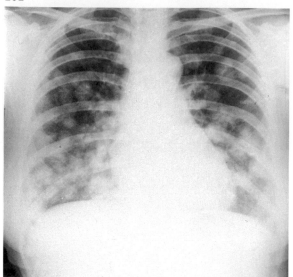

102

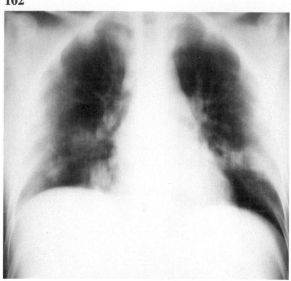

101   Secondary deposits from a carcinoma of the colon. Well-demarcated cannon ball 'shadows' are present throughout both lung fields. Metastatic carcinoma is the commonest cause. They may also reflect tuberculosis, lymphoma, rheumatoid lung, sarcoidosis, histoplasmosis, coccidioidomycosis, hydatid cysts, Wegener's granulomatosis and septicaemic pneumonia. At least two of the nodules should exceed 1 cm in diameter. Smaller sized multiple nodules are classified as diffuse disseminated miliary or reticulonodular infiltration (see Chapter 7).

102   Multiple pulmonary nodules with cavitation in Hodgkin's disease. (Tomogram)

103

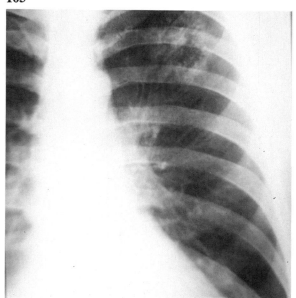

103   Calcification in metastases from osteogenic sarcoma. Metastatic nodules from ovary, breast, testis or chondrosarcoma may also calcify.

7 Diffuse interstitial or miliary patterns

Diffuse shadowing may be caused by widespread inflammatory or infiltrative involvement of the alveolar walls, blood vessels, lymphatics, bronchioles and the connective tissue framework.

Bilateral interstitial shadowing may be described as reticular, fishnet, honeycomb or alternatively as diffuse miliary or micronodular shadows.

The radiographic appearance is composed of large numbers of minute overlapping nodules, each up to 5 mm in diameter. The patterns may vary.

A classification of mixed diffuse miliary or interstitial patterns of disease indicates that widely differing disorders produce confusingly similar radiographic patterns.

This chapter on the radiographic patterns of disease should be read with Chapter 18 where interstitial lung diseases are described in more detail.

1 Infections

Virus
Influenza
Varicella
Smallpox
Measles
Q fever
Cytomegalo
Psittacosis
Mycoplasma
Legionnaires'

Parasite
Pneumocystis
Schistosoma
Microfilaria

Mycobacteria
– tuberculosis
– atypical

Bacterial
Gram-negative bacilli
Staphylococcus

Fungal
Histoplasma
Coccidioides
Blastomyces (South American)
Candida
Cryptococcus
Aspergillus

104

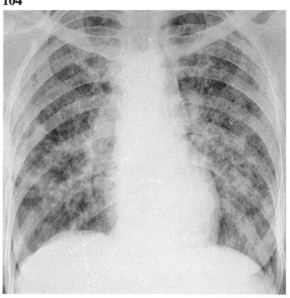

104 Widely disseminated micronodular shadows in miliary tuberculosis. This appearance with 2 to 5 mm well-defined and widely distributed nodular shadows is typical, but not exclusive, in miliary tuberculosis.

2 Pneumoconiosis

Silicosis
Coal miners'
Asbestosis
Beryllium
Talc
Graphite
Aluminium (bauxite)
Silo fillers'

6 Fibrosing alveolitis

Desquamative alveolitis
Rheumatoid arthritis
Systemic lupus
Systemic sclerosis
(Scleroderma)
Neurofibromatosis
Dermatomyositis
Polymyositis

Drugs

Gold
Nitrofurantoin
Busulphan
Methotrexate
Bleomycin

3 Allergic alveolitis

Farmers' lung   Suberosis
Bagassosis   Detergent
Air conditioning   Pituitary snuff
Bird fancier lung   Cheese washer
Maple bark   Malt worker
Sequoia tree   Mushroom worker

7 Autoimmune disease

Sjogren's syndrome
Fibrosing alveolitis

4 Malignancy

Alveolar cell carcinoma

Metastases < haematogenous / lymphatic

Leukaemia
Hodgkin's disease

Drugs

Bleomycin

Methotrexate
Busulphan

8 Miscellaneous

Sarcoidosis
Histiocytosis X
(eosinophilic granuloma)
Thesaurosis
Alveolar proteinosis
Macroglobulinaemia

5 Cardiovascular disease

Mitral stenosis
Haemosiderosis
Goodpasture's syndrome
Talc emboli

105a

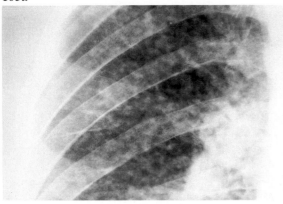

105a Coal workers' pneumoconiosis with interstitial miliary nodular shadows. Miliary tuberculosis has a similar appearance.

105b

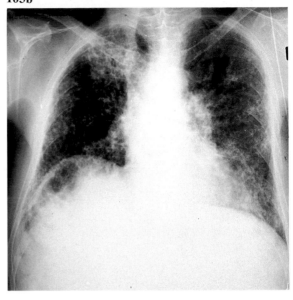

105b Scleroderma lung with 'honeycomb' like cystic spaces and nodular shadows (see page 174).

106

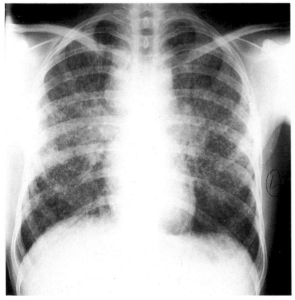

106 Miliary mottling with hilar and right paratracheal lymphadenopathy. The radiological diagnosis was of tuberculosis or sarcoidosis. It turned out to be the latter.

107

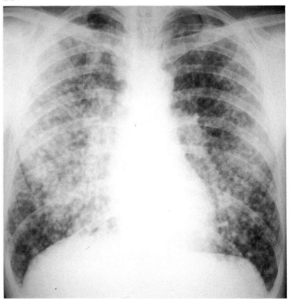

107 Miliary nodular shadows from metastatic adeno-carcinoma of pancreas in a symptom-free man aged 52 years.

51

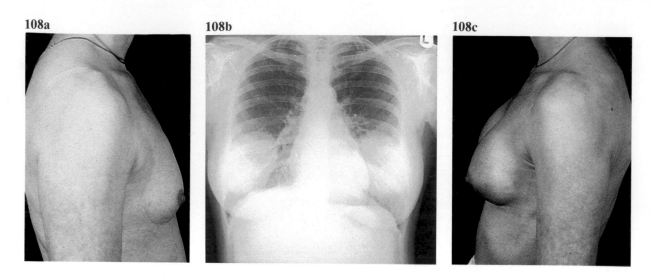

Extra-pulmonary radiographic shadowing

Confusing radiographic shadows may be produced by soft tissues, clothing or artefacts. There are many possible causes.

108a, b and c   Breast shadows after cosmetic mammary augmentation. Bilateral opaque silicone filled prosthetic implants are seen on the xray. **108a** and **108c** show the presurgical and postsurgical state. The radiographic opacities from the prostheses seldom cause diagnostic confusion but may obscure lesions in the underlying lung.

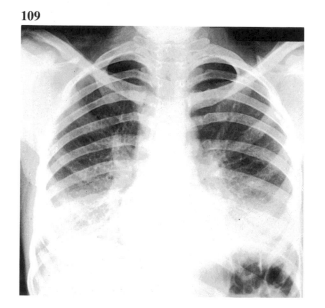

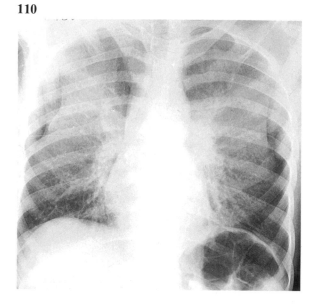

109   Breast shadows – bilateral lower zone shadowing. In adolescent girls the breasts are often relatively radio-opaque, in spite of their small size. The soft tissue radiographic shadow may simulate consolidation or bilateral basal lung fibrosis.

110   Breast shadows (same patient as **109**). This xray was taken after the patient had elevated the breasts. The normal lung bases are clearly seen. A lateral radiograph would also localise the breast shadows.

8 Consolidation

Consolidation of the lung occurs when alveolar air has been replaced by fluid, exudate or cells. Airlessness without shrinkage occurs in all types of pneumonia, in pulmonary oedema, when bleeding occurs into the alveoli, or when the alveoli are filled by neoplastic cells. The radiograph shows dense homogeneous opacification occupying the normal position of a lobe or segment. When consolidation occurs in association with atelectasis, the possibility of malignant bronchial obstruction should be considered. This chapter is illustrated by examples of consolidation in which associated collapse is minimal.

111a

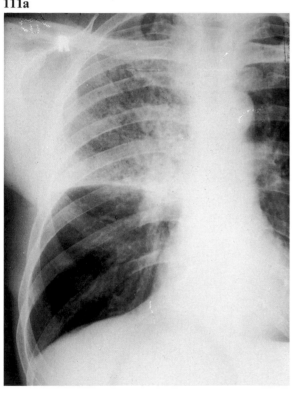

111a Right upper lobe consolidation caused by pneumococcal pneumonia. Consolidation of the whole right upper lobe is commonly seen in children. The homogeneous shadow extends from the apex downwards to end in a well-defined inferior margin at the horizontal fissure, which in this example is normally placed.

111b

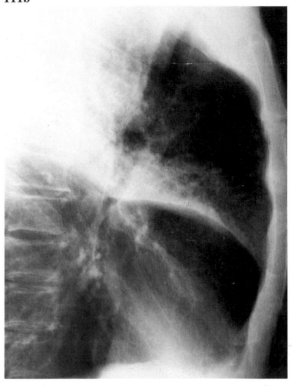

111b Right upper lobe consolidation. The lateral film shows a well-defined posterior and inferior border corresponding to the oblique and horizontal fissures. Consolidation involves the posterior and anterior segments.

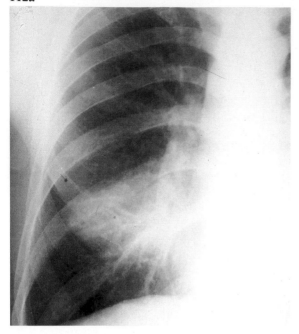

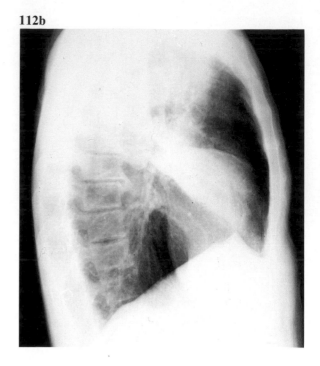

112a Consolidation in right middle lobe. The right heart border is indistinct because of the overlying consolidation causing the 'silhouette sign'. This sign is based upon the observation that an intrathoracic opacity lying against the border of the heart, diaphragm or great vessels will obliterate that border.

112b Consolidation in right middle lobe. The lateral film shows the wedge-shaped area of consolidation overlying the heart bounded by the horizontal and oblique fissures.

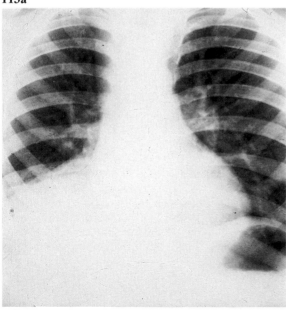

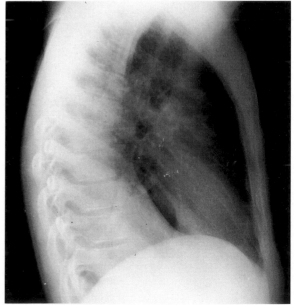

113a Consolidation of right lower lobe. The diaphragm and right cardiac border are obscured.

113b Consolidation in right lower lobe. The lateral film localises the consolidation. There is a slight loss of volume.

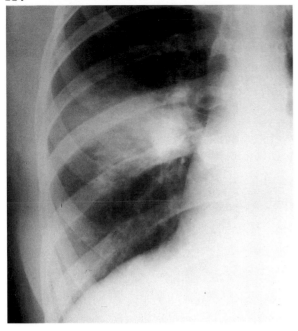

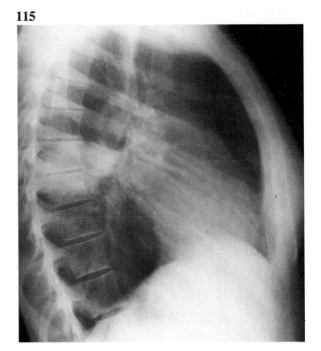

114 Consolidation in apical segment of right lower lobe. The PA film shows a circumscribed homogeneous area in the right mid-zone which could be caused by involvement of the lateral segment of the right middle lobe, or of the apical segment of the right lower lobe.

115 Consolidation in apical segment of right lower lobe. The lateral film localises the consolidation to the apical segment of the right lower lobe.

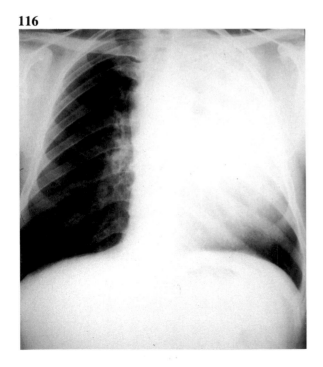

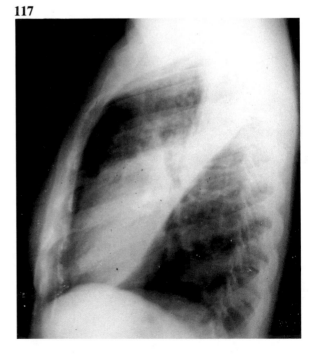

116 Consolidation of left upper lobe with involvement of the lingula. The PA film shows a dense homogeneous opacity continuous with the left heart border.

117 Consolidation of the left upper lobe. The lateral film shows a well-defined fissure with consolidation in the posterior segment of the left upper lobe and lingula.

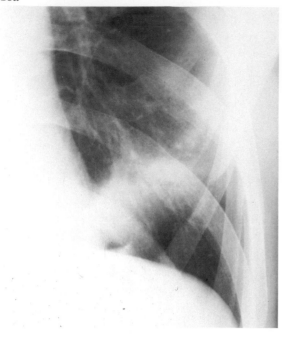

118a Consolidation in lingula. The shadowing lies against the left heart border.

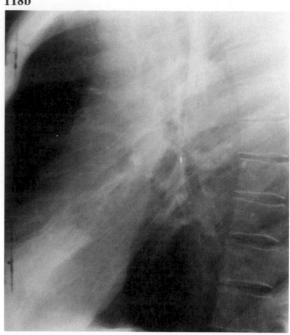

118b Consolidation in lingula. The lateral film localises the consolidation.

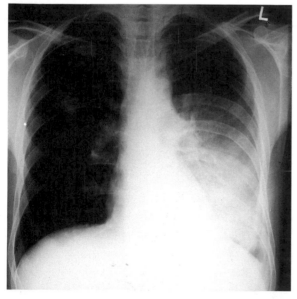

119a   Consolidation in left lower lobe. The diaphragm is obscured by the consolidation.

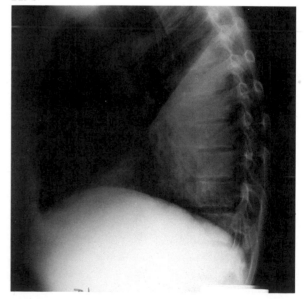

119b   Consolidation in left lower lobe. This lobar consolidation was due to pneumococcal pneumonia.

9 Atelectasis

Atelectasis is a loss of volume of a lobe or segment, usually accompanied by increased radiographic opacification of the involved lung. It is usually due to obstruction, resulting from intrinsic block of a bronchus by a carcinoma or foreign body or extrinsic compression when encircling glands compress the bronchus. Obstructive collapse may occur due to fibrosis and chronic inflammation following pneumonia. Postoperative atelectasis of the lower lobe segments is common and predisposes to infection.

120

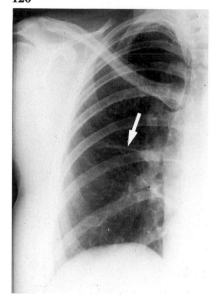

120   Atelectasis of anterior segment of the right upper lobe.

121

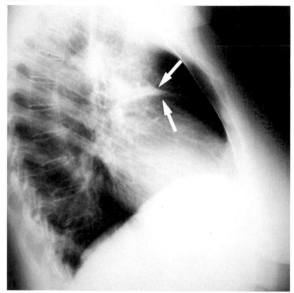

121   Atelectasis of anterior segment of the right upper lobe. Lateral view.

122

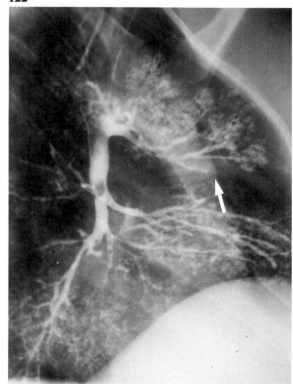

122   Atelectasis of anterior segment of the right upper lobe. The bronchogram shows narrowing of the segmental bronchus caused by fibrosis after pneumonia.

123

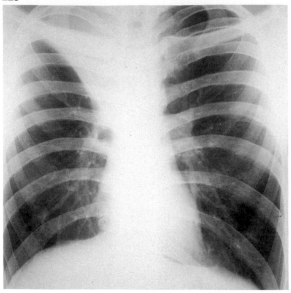

123 Partial collapse of right upper lobe. The lung re-expanded when a mucus plug was aspirated from the bronchus of this asthmatic patient.

124

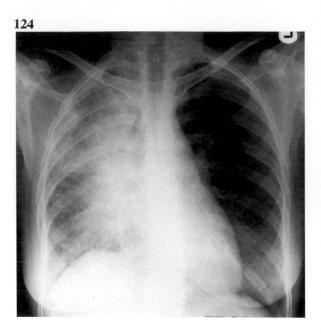

124 Collapse of right upper lobe caused by a proximal small cell carcinoma. Diffuse shadowing and elevation of the right diaphragm are visible.

125

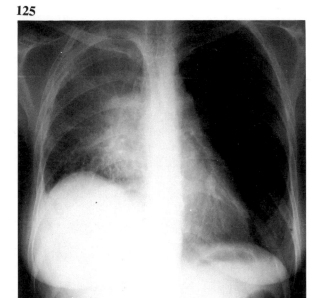

125 Collapse of right upper lobe. Five weeks later the diaphragm is more elevated and the shadowing less apparent. There is a small right pleural effusion.

126

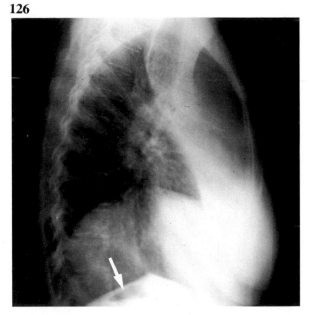

126 Collapse of the right upper lobe. The lateral view shows displacement of the oblique fissure upwards and forwards to cross the thoracic spine at the level of the first thoracic vertebra. A gastric air bubble is present below the left diaphragm (arrowed).

127

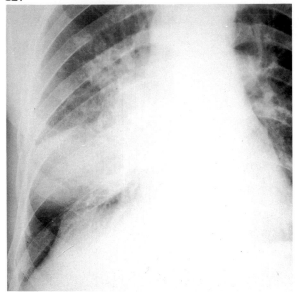

127 Partial collapse of right middle lobe. The horizontal fissure is pulled down.

128

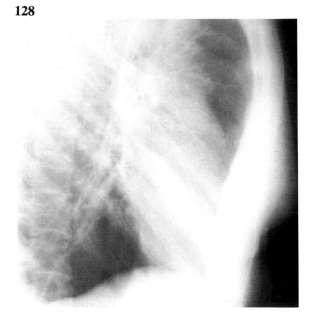

128 Partial collapse of right middle lobe. Lateral view shows a narrow homogeneous shadow lying over the heart shadow.

129

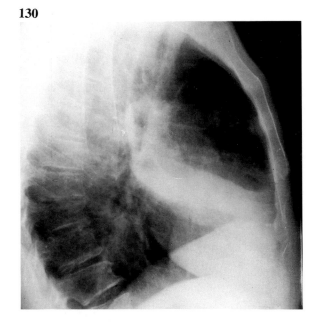

129 Complete collapse of right middle lobe. The right heart border is blurred. Note the well defined nipple shadow.

130

130 Complete collapse of right middle lobe. Lateral view.

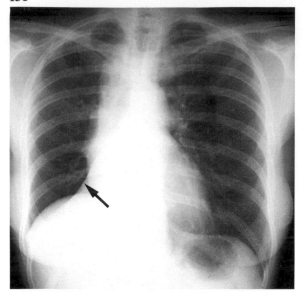

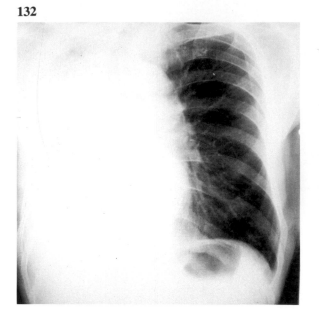

131 Collapse of right lower lobe. The triangular shadow at the right cardiophrenic angle continues towards the costophrenic angle.

132 Collapse of right lung caused by an obstruction of the main bronchus by an oat-cell carcinoma. The trachea and heart are deviated to the right towards the side of the collapse.

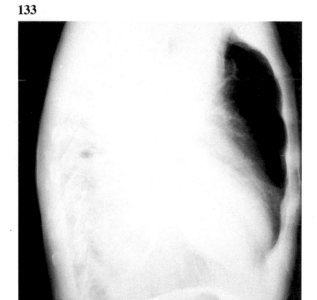

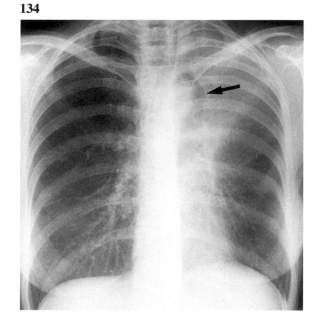

133 Collapse of right lung. Lateral view of **132**. The anterior mediastinal translucency is caused by the over-inflated left lung.

134 Collapse of left upper lobe. Bronchostenosis of the left upper lobe often includes the lingula. This PA view shows a hazy homogeneous opacity in the left upper zone obliterating the left heart border. The right lung is herniated across the midline (arrowed).

135

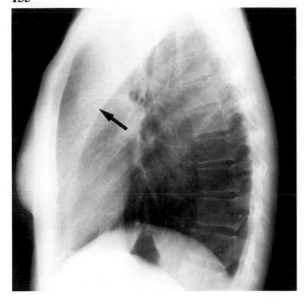

135   Collapse of left upper lobe. The lateral film shows upward and forward displacement of the interlobar fissure (arrowed).

136

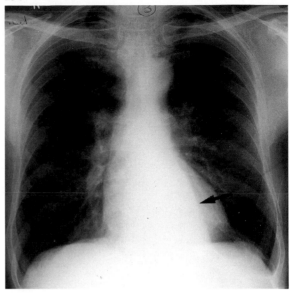

136   Collapse of left lower lobe seen as a dense shadow behind the heart with a well-defined left margin sloping downwards and outwards. The left hilum is displaced downwards.

137

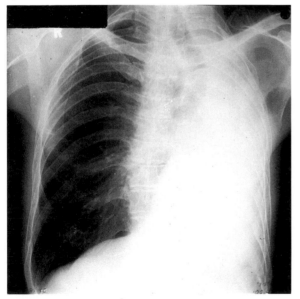

137   Complete collapse of left lung. The mediastinum and trachea are markedly deviated to the left and the diaphragm is obscured.

138

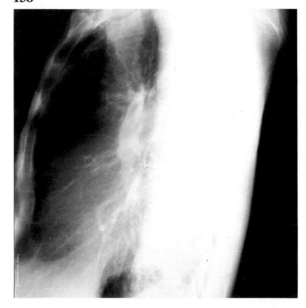

138   Complete collapse of left lung. The lateral view shows a large radiolucent area anterior to the heart as a result of compensatory expansion to the left of the aerated right lung. The left diaphragm is elevated and the collapsed lung lies posterior.

10 Hypertransradiancy

The normal radiographic appearance of the lung is a composite shadow picture comprising pulmonary vessels and soft tissue shadows of the body wall muscle and ribs. Bilateral hypertransradiancy (hypertranslucency) is difficult to see but a local loss of lung density may be detected by comparison with other areas of normal lung. Comparisons can also be made between equivalent matching areas in both lungs.

Hypertransradiancy	Possible causes
Extrathoracic (usually unilateral)	Absent female breast Absent pectoral muscle Severe scoliosis Increased density of other side Rotation of body
Intrathoracic Extrapulmonary	Pneumothorax Diaphragmatic hernia
Intrathoracic Intrapulmonary (unilateral)	Obstructive emphysema (foreign body, neoplasm) Macleod's syndrome Bronchogenic cyst or bulla Post-lobectomy
Intrathoracic Intrapulmonary (bilateral)	Simple emphysema Cystic bronchiectasis

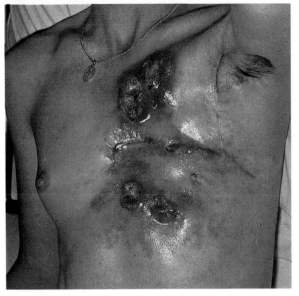

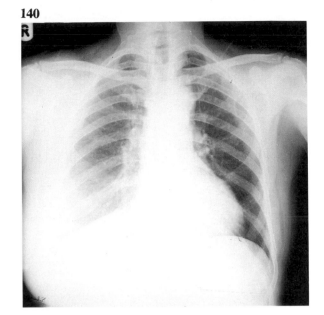

139 and 140 Mastectomy with recurrent local tumour (139). An example of a chest-wall abnormality causing radiographic hypertransradiancy of the lung field. The xray taken three years previously shows the difference in radiodensity produced by the loss of soft tissue between the right and left lower lung fields (**140**).

141

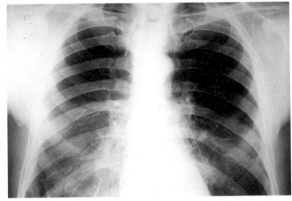

141 Early obstructive emphysema of left upper lobe. A comparison of both upper zones shows fewer vessels on the left.

142

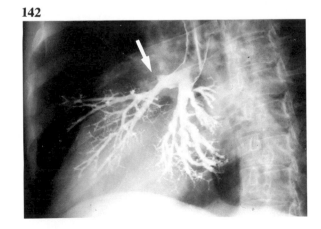

142 Bronchogram of 141 – lateral oblique view. Filling of the left lower lobe and lingula is normal but a carcinoma is causing obstruction at the origin of the left upper lobe bronchus. A ball-valve mechanism allows air to enter on inspiration but it is retained during expiration. Collapse of the lobe usually follows.

143

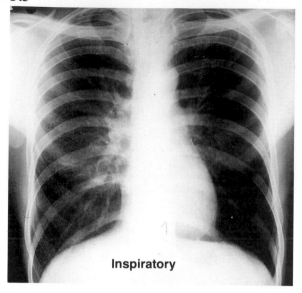

Inspiratory

144

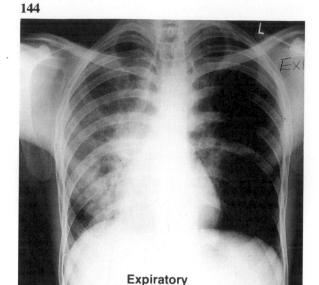

Expiratory

143 Macleod's syndrome – inspiratory film. The left lung is hypertransradiant as a result of hypoplasia of the pulmonary artery and peripheral vessels. The primary abnormality is bronchiolitis with airway obstruction and the affected lung has little if any function. The bronchi have a normal number of branches but a diminished complement of alveoli suggesting alveolar injury before eight years of age; the total adult number of alveoli develop at about this age.

144 Macleod's syndrome – expiratory film. The mediastinal structures are now deviated to the right as a consequence of air trapping in the left lung.
Lung damage probably occurs during infection with measles, whooping cough or other childhood respiratory infections. Inevitably the hypoplastic lung is the most damaged, although at necropsy similar patchy damage is often found in the radiographically normal lung.

145

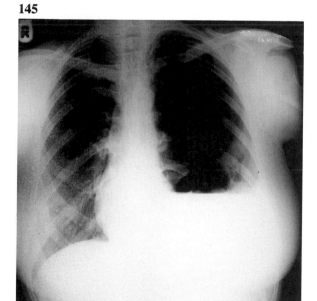

146

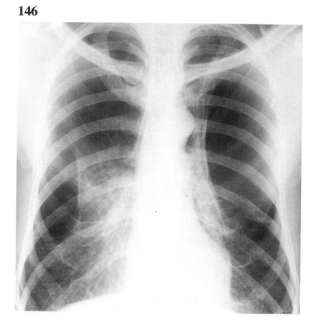

145 Fluid level in huge bulla which was mistaken for a tension pneumothorax because of the mediastinal shift to the right.

146 Bilateral bullae. Both bullae were removed with significant improvement in lung function. Note the considerable hyperinflation with low flat diaphragm.

147

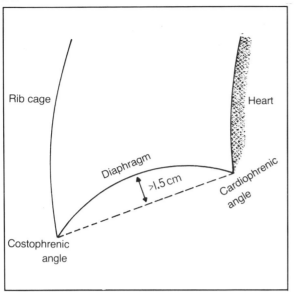

147 Measuring the diaphragm curve. The costophrenic and cardiophrenic angles are joined by a line drawn between them. A vertical line drawn from this to the highest point on the curve of the diaphragm is normally in excess of 1.5 cm.

148

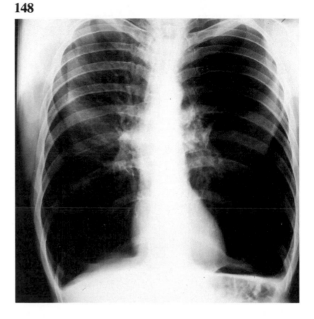

148 Hypertransradiant lung caused by severe emphysema. The diaphragm is low and flat and the prominent right upper zone 'marker vessels' contrast with the few narrowed vessels elsewhere.

Radiographic features of widespread emphysema

The radiograph correlates poorly with functional changes in moderate emphysema and even severe structural changes may not produce significant radiographic abnormalities.

The following features are typical of severe pan lobular (panacinar) emphysema.

Hyperinflation
1 Low diaphragms. The right diaphragm lies below the anterior end of the 6th rib.
2 Flat diaphragms (see **147**).
3 Visible phrenocostal muscle attachments.
4 Deep PA diameter on lateral chest xray.
5 Increased retrosternal transradiancy on lateral chest xray.
6 Bullae or hypertransradiant bullous areas.

Cardiovascular changes
1 Peripheral lung vessels diminished in size and number.
2 Prominent hilar vessels.
3 Narrow vertical heart.

149

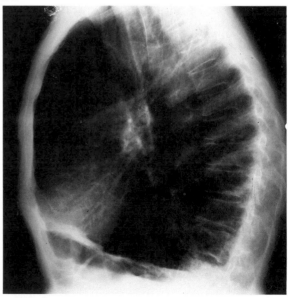

149 Hypertransradiant lung. The lateral film shows large anterior translucency with deep posteroanterior measurement (same patient as **148**).

11 Calcification

Dense opacities are commonly caused by calcification. The size, shape, position and relationship to adjacent structures may point to the cause of the calcium deposits.

Identification of calcium in a solitary pulmonary nodule is of great importance in management and diagnosis (see page 42). Central calcification is a reliable sign that the lesion is benign; usually from healed fungal or tuberculous infections. Calcification at the periphery usually indicates a benign lesion, but rarely may represent a pre-existing healed granuloma engulfed by a neoplasm arising in a lung scar.

Peripheral 'egg-shell' calcification of lymph nodes is a feature of sarcoidosis and silicosis.

Calcification in multiple pulmonary nodules is also commonly caused by healed fungal or tuberculous infections. Rarely multiple pulmonary metastases from osteosarcoma, thyroid, ovary, testis or breast may calcify.

Unilateral pleural calcification occurs as linear or oval plaques on the diaphragm, or as visceral pleura on the lateral chest wall. Haemothorax, empyema or tuberculosis are common causes.

Bilateral pleural calcified plaques on the parietal pleura and diaphragm may signify asbestosis or other pneumoconiosis (talc, bakelite, mica). Damaged heart valves and atherosclerotic blood vessels may calcify, as may hilar lymph nodes and the lung parenchyma.

Pleural calcification

150

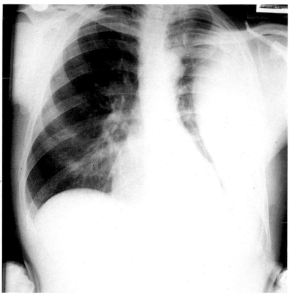

150 Old calcified artificial pneumothorax. A dense homogeneous shadow occupies most of the left lung field. This rare occurrence sometimes follows intrathoracic bleeding induced by repeated artificial pneumothoraces.

151

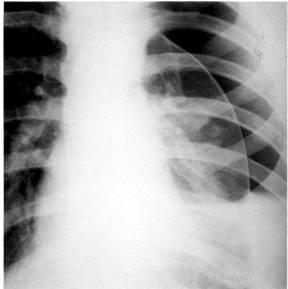

151 Haemopneumothorax occurring in a patient whose pulmonary tuberculosis was treated by repeated artificial pneumothoraces.

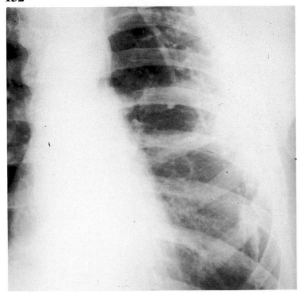

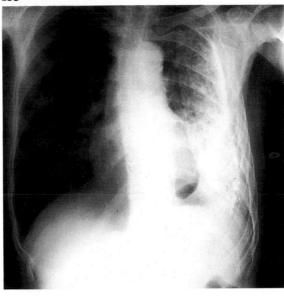

152   Haemopneumothorax. Thirty years later there is extensive pleural calcification (same patient as **151**).

153   Pleural calcification caused by an old tuberculous pleural effusion. The left lung is shrunken and encased by thickened calcified pleura.

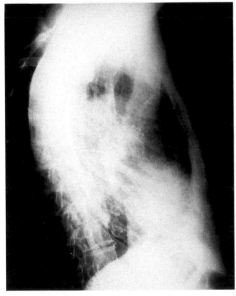

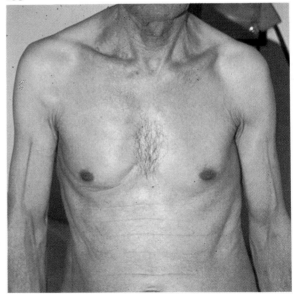

154   Pleural calcification. Lateral view of **153**.

155   Pleural calcification. The left chest is flattened and the spine curved, left shoulder and nipple drooping as a consequence of the contracted left lung. Remember the aphorism flattening of the chest is often due to underlying lung fibrosis (same patient as **153**).

156

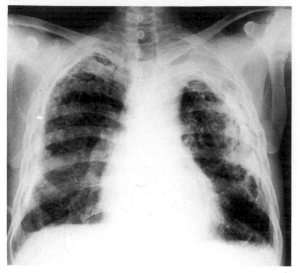

157

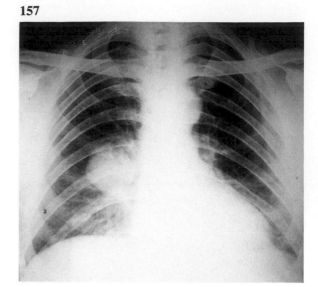

156 Bilateral pleural calcification after tuberculosis. There was no history of occupational exposure to asbestos. Note that the calcium is deposited near the inner surface of the greatly thickened pleura. This results in a clear linear radiolucent space between the calcification and the bony thorax on tangential projection.

157 Benign hamartoma. This patient had a right pneumonectomy for a suspected carcinoma. The large mass adjacent to the right hilum proved to be a benign hamartoma.

158

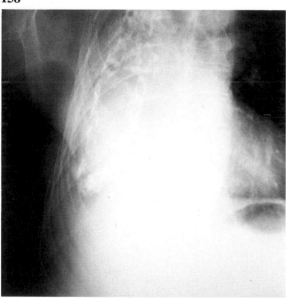

159

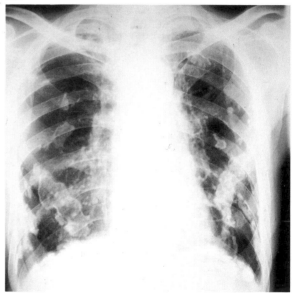

158 Pleural calcification. Twelve years after pneumonectomy. A large irregular area of pleural calcification resulted from troublesome postoperative bleeding into the pleural space.

159 Extensive parietal pleural calcification from asbestos exposure in a shipbuilding worker. Bilateral diaphragmatic calcification is extensive and characteristic. It may herald a subsequent mesothelioma.

160

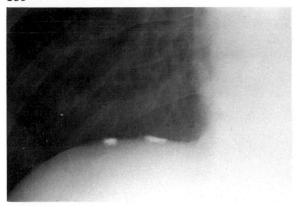

160 Calcification of the diaphragmatic pleura caused by asbestos exposure.

161 Irregular pleural shadowing provides a 'holly-leaf' appearance typical of asbestos exposure. The calcification occurs on the parietal pleura.

161

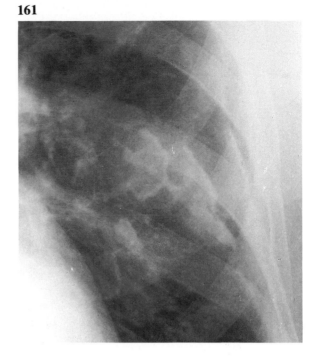

Hilar calcification

162

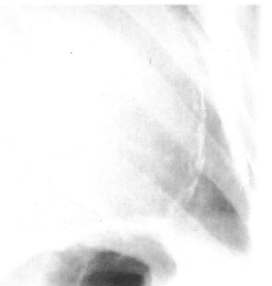

162 Calcified healing. This patient had pulmonary tuberculosis in childhood and a large anterior myocardial infarction in middle age. The two unrelated lesions healed with calcification.

163

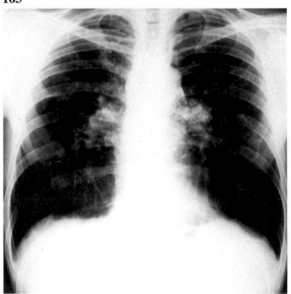

163 Bilateral hilar calcification caused by sarcoidosis. This patient had chronic sarcoidosis with persistent hypercalciuria. Calcified hilar lymph nodes are almost always caused by tuberculosis but may also be noted in silicosis and chronic sarcoidosis.

Calcification in blood vessels

164

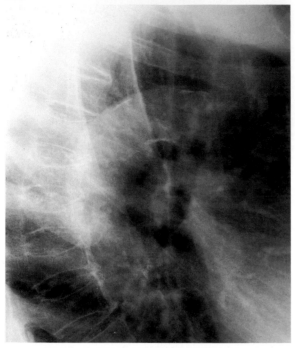

165

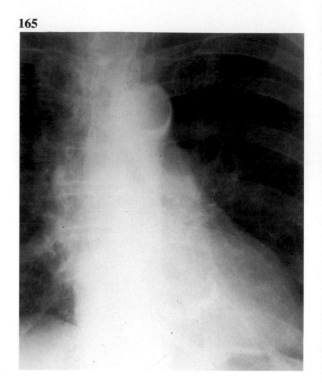

164 and 165   Calcified aortic arch is commonplace with ageing.

166

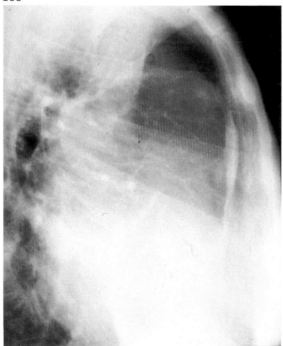

166   Calcified syphilitic ascending aorta.

167

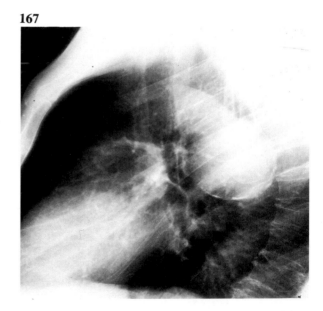

167   Calcification in a traumatic aortic aneurysm which resulted from a road traffic accident.

Pulmonary calcification

168

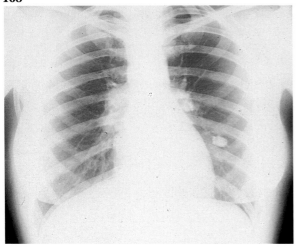

168 Healed tuberculous 'primary complex' (Ghon focus). There is a dense localised area of calcification in the left mid-zone and in the draining left hilar lymph node.

169

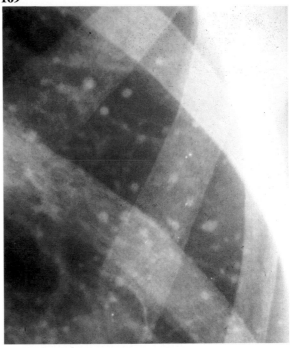

169 Discrete dense shadows about 2 mm in size may follow haemorrhagic chickenpox pneumonia, particularly in the adult. The dense calcification usually appears within two years of acute severe adult infection. Similar 1 mm to 2 mm circular calcified shadows may follow histoplasmosis (see page 120).

170

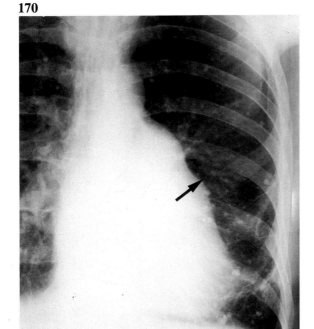

170 Dense uniform opacities caused by ectopic bone formation may occur in mitral stenosis or rarely after acute rheumatic fever without valve disease. Note the characteristic appearance of the cardiac silhouette which accompanies severe mitral stenosis. The left atrium and left atrial appendage (arrowed) are enlarged.

12 Tubes, band and line shadows

These common radiographic shadows are all essentially linear, varying in width from barely discernible lines of 1 mm to 2 mm to well-defined bands of 1 cm to 2 cm in width.

Tubular shadows are evident when a couple of line shadows are closely parallel. The diagnostic challenge constantly facing us is whether these shadows reflect diseases or normal structures and artefacts.

171

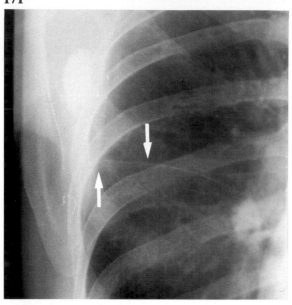

171 The horizontal fissure may appear as a line shadow on a PA xray.

172

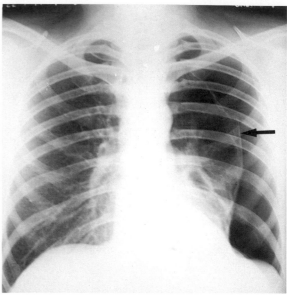

172 A fine linear shadow of visceral pleura marks the lung edge of a pneumothorax.

173

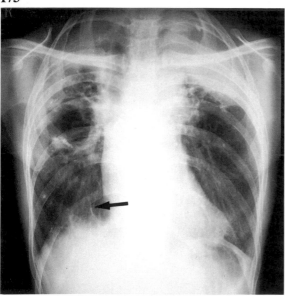

173 Vertical line shadow extending upwards from the diaphragm is due to indrawn visceral pleura.

174

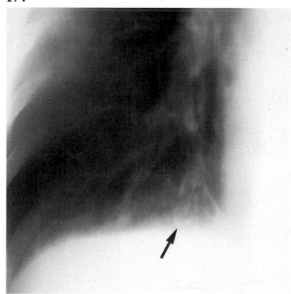

174 Tubular 'tram line' shadows caused by localised bronchiectasis in lower lobe. The bronchial walls are thickened and dilated.

175

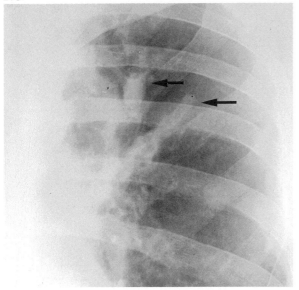

175 Band-like and tubular shadows. Two dilated upper-lobe bronchi are filled with secretions producing a V-shaped band shadow. Tubular or ring shadows of air-filled, dilated, thick-walled bronchi are seen adjacent to the hilum. The diagnosis was allergic bronchopulmonary aspergillosis.

176

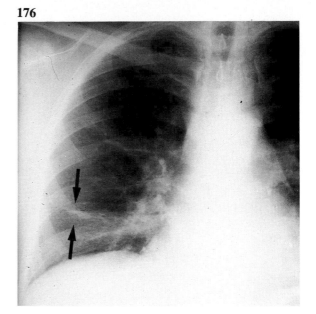

176 Horizontal linear shadows (discoid atelectasis). These shadows represent atelectasis caused by obstruction of medium-sized bronchi, developing when diaphragmatic movement is limited: postoperative pain, pleurisy, rib fracture and pulmonary embolism.

177

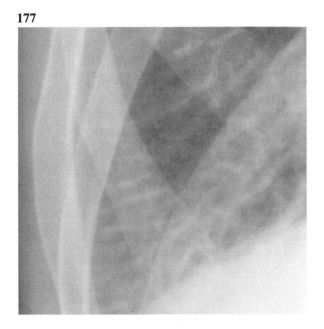

177 Kerley 'B' septal line shadows at the right lung base in a patient with left ventricular failure. The fine transverse lines represent oedema and thickening in the interlobular septa, and appear as horizontal lines 1 cm to 3 cm in length and 1 mm to 2 mm in width located perpendicular to a pleural surface. These transient lines are caused by raised pulmonary venous pressure. They may persist if the lymphatic channels are obstructed by tumour, choked by dust particles in pneumoconiosis, or thickened by fibrosing alveolitis.

178

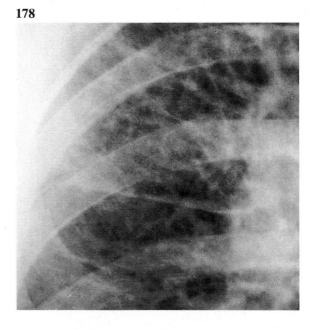

178 Kerley 'A' lines reflect thickened intercommunicating lymphatics, and appear as thin, non-branching lines several inches in length extending out from the hilum. These persistent 'A' lines were caused by lymphangitis carcinomatosa. Transient 'A' lines may be seen when left ventricular failure develops rapidly or in pulmonary oedema caused by drug hypersensitivity.

13 Apical lesions

It is difficult to disentangle the apex because of the overlying first and second ribs and clavicle, so tomography and lordotic views are invaluable in recognising normal structures, artefacts and disease. Apical lesions lie within the circle of the first rib; subapical lesions lie between the circle of the first and second ribs.

Normal structures and artefacts	Apical and subapical lesions
Azygos lobe (right)	Pleural cap fibrosis
Cervical rib	Pancoast superior sulcus tumour
Sternomastoid muscle	Tuberculosis
Lock of hair	Mycoses
Clothing	Aspergillosis
Retrosternal thyroid	Mycetoma
Subclavian artery	Neurofibroma
	Ankylosing spondylitis
	Irradiation fibrosis
	Alveolar cell carcinoma
	Metastases
	Cysts, blebs, bullae

179

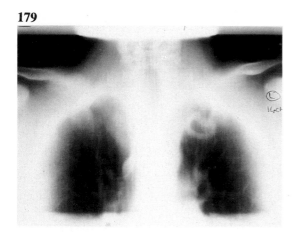

180

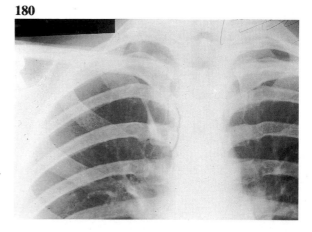

179 Apical cavity caused by tuberculosis, best seen on tomography.

180 Accessory lobe of azygos vein. The hairline shadow extends from the apical pleura to a comma-like expansion near the hilum. The line shadow represents a double layer of visceral parietal pleura which encloses the abnormally placed azygos vein.

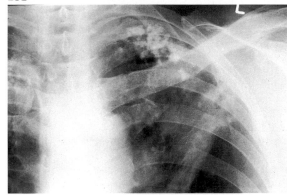

181 Bilateral apical and subapical calcification from healed pulmonary tuberculosis.

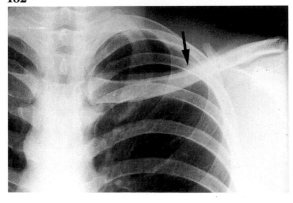

182 Companion shadows above the clavicle. A 2mm to 3mm wide companion shadow is often seen running parallel to the upper border of the clavicle. This shadow is lost if the supraclavicular lymph nodes are enlarged. It is caused by the fold of skin and subcutaneous tissue lying horizontally above the bone, which represents a considerable thickness of tissue to the xray beam.

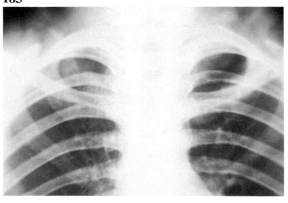

183 Hair or clothing may simulate an apical lesion.

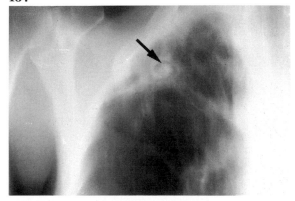

184 A small aspergilloma lying within a subapical cavity in the right lung. Chronic lung cavities, irrespective of their aetiology, may be colonised by fungal spores.

75

14 Pneumonia

After cardiovascular disease and malignant neoplasms, respiratory infection is the next most common cause of death worldwide. Acute respiratory tract infections account for 57 deaths per 100,000 population in well-developed countries compared with 76 in less well-developed areas. The three killers worldwide are pneumonia, influenza and bronchitis.

A classification of pneumonias is given in the tables below. The commonest pathogens found in sputum or transtracheal aspirates are the pneumococcus in about one-half of patients, Haemophilus influenzae in one-quarter, Neisseriae in one-tenth, and less often Staphylococcus aureus and Staphylococcus viridans.

However, a histopathological classification of pneumonia is of little value to the clinician in deciding about appropriate treatment. History, physical examination, chest xray, measurement of total and differential white-blood cell count and in some cases immediate Gram stain of sputum usually suffice.

In most cases the initial therapeutic decision will be correct and the patient will show signs of substantial recovery within 48 to 72 hours. Further measures may be necessary in those patients who have not improved. Sputum cultures often yield upper airway flora rather than the causative organism. Purer cultures may be sought by performing direct lung or transtracheal puncture or obtaining lung washings through a sterile catheter at fibreoptic bronchoscopy.

Other possible infective agents disregarded at presentation should be looked for at this stage. Acute serological studies for viral, mycoplasma, rickettsial or legionella infections may be useful. In the immuno-compromised patient coliforms, Pneumocystis, Pseudomonas aeruginosa, M. tuberculosis or pathogenic fungi may be present.

Finally, structural factors which may delay resolution, such as bronchial blockage by carcinoma, should be considered.

Table: Classification of pneumonia.

Infections	Hypersensitivity
Gram-positive cocci	
Gram-negative bacilli	Chemical
Mycobacteria	
Yeasts and fungi	Aspiration
Virus	
Rickettsial	
Miscellaneous	

Table: Respiratory infections.

Family	Pathogenic organism Member	Isolation from	Blood test	Treatment	Remarks
Gram-positive cocci	Streptococcus	Sputum Blood	Leucocytosis	Benzylpenicillin G or amoxycillin or a	Consider polyvalent pneumococcal vaccine for the immunosuppressed, the elderly and bronchitics
	– pneumoniae		Specific poly-saccharide in blood and body fluids	cephalosporin or erythromycin	
	– pyogenes	Sputum Blood		– do –	Usually found complicating influenza and other virus infections
	Staphylococcus aureus	Sputum Blood	Leucocytosis	Benzylpenicillin G or flucloxacillin or a cephalosporin or erythromycin	Complicating virus infections, cystic fibrosis, immunodeficient infants

Table: Respiratory infections.

Pathogenic organism Family	Member	Isolation from	Blood test	Treatment	Remarks
Gram-negative bacilli	Klebsiella pneumoniae (Friedlander)	Sputum Blood		Cefoxitin	Necrotising upper lobe pneumonia with red-currant jelly sputum, pleurisy and abscesses particularly in the immunodeficient and alcoholic
	Haemophilus – influenzae	Sputum Blood Cerebrospinal fluid Pleural fluid	Anti-type B antibodies	Amoxycillin ± chloramphenicol	Epiglottitis necessitates tracheostomy
	Bordetella pertussis	Pernasal swab Cough plate	Leucocytosis Lymphocytosis	Erythromycin or chloramphenicol	Consider hyperimmune human gamma globulin in the unimmunised
	Pasteurella – tularensis	Sputum Blood Body fluids	Serum agglutinins	Streptomycin ± tetracycline	Xray shows oval lesions with hilar adenopathy and pleurisy
	Bacteroides fragilis and fusobacteria	Sputum Pleural fluid Transtracheal aspiration Bronchoscopy Blood		Metronidazole or cefoxitin	Pulmonary necrosis, foul-smelling sputum associated empyema. May be aspirated from peritonsillar abscess
Mycobacteria	– tuberculosis	Sputum		Rifampicin Isoniazid Ethambutol Streptomycin Pyrazinamide	Particularly in the immunodeficient elderly and certain ethnic groups
	– atypical	Sputum		– do –	Usually white males over 45 years old with pre-existing chronic pulmonary disease
Actinomycetes	A-Israeli	Pus, sinus or empyema track		Benzylpenicillin G	Pneumonia with empyema and sinus
	Nocardia	Sputum, pus, bronchoscopy, sinus		Sulphonamide + streptomycin	Particularly in the immunodeficient, including alveolar proteinosis
Miscellaneous	Mycoplasma pneumoniae	Sputum Throat washings	Normal leucocyte count Cold agglutinins Mycoplasma CFT	Tetracycline or erythromycin	Usually accompanies myringitis with bulla on tympanic membrane
	Legionella pneumophila	Lung, sputum Pleural exudate Sputum Transtracheal aspirate	Normal leucocyte count Serum fluorescent antibodies	Rifampicin or erythromycin	More frequent in male town-dwellers
	Chlamydia psittaci	Sputum Blood	Psittacosis CFT Normal leucocyte count	Tetracycline	Contracted from birds. A penicillin-resistant pneumonia
	Pneumocystis carinii	Sputum Transbronchial or open lung biopsy	±leucocytosis ±eosinophilia Oxygen desaturation	Co-trimoxazole	Particularly in the immunosuppressed recipients of transplants
	Coxiella burneti	Special laboratories only	Complement-fixing and agglutinating antibodies	Tetracycline or chloramphenicol	Penicillin-resistant pneumonia. Contracted from sheep and cattle
Virus	Influenza	Sputum Throat washings	Serum antibodies	Oxygen therapy Antibiotics to control secondary bacterial pneumonia	Complicated by secondary bacterial bronchopneumonia

Pneumococcal pneumonia

The pneumococcus was first recognised by Pasteur in 1880 when he recovered it from sputum. We now recognise 83 serotypes, 14 of which are included in a new polyvalent capsular polysaccharide vaccine available for protection of the immunodeficient from pneumococcal infection.

Streptococcus pneumoniae is a common cause of lobar consolidation especially in previously healthy adult males.

The typical features are of rigor, fever, chest pain and cough with blood-stained sputum.

185

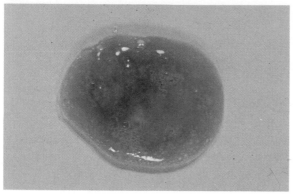

185 Rusty red mucopurulent sputum specimen in pneumococcal pneumonia. Sputum may be initially scanty or absent, later becoming purulent.

186

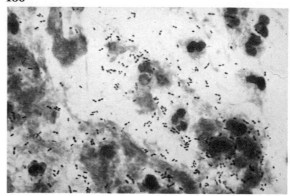

186 Gram-positive, lancet-shaped diplococci in association with polymorphonuclear leucocytes in sputum specimen. *(Gram stain ×1000)*

187

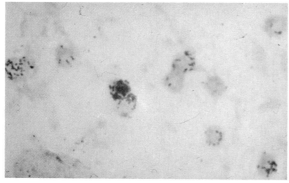

187 Cerebrospinal fluid containing S. pneumoniae and pus cells in purulent pneumococcal meningitis. Bacteraemia is evident in about one-quarter of patients with bacterial pneumonia. Ideally, blood cultures should be part of the investigative routine. *(Gram stain ×1000)*

188

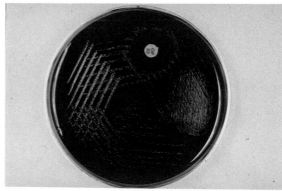

188 Culture of pneumococci on blood agar medium. Typical colonies are flat with raised margins, sometimes likened to 'draughtsmen'.

The colonies are surrounded by a zone of green discolouration or alpha haemolysis caused by destruction of the red blood cells in the culture medium.

The growth of S. pneumoniae is inhibited by optochin (ethyl hydriecuprein hydrochloride) which assists bacteriological confirmation (optochin disc = OP10).

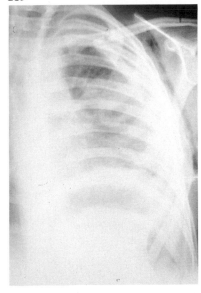

189 Empyema may complicate pneumococcal pneumonia, especially if treatment is delayed. Its presence is indicated by continued fever, persistent leucocytosis and pleural effusion.

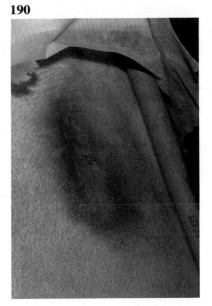

190 Empyema. Untreated empyema may spontaneously rupture through the chest wall. Note this abscess pointing at the initial old drainage site. The second intercostal tube was inserted too high and failed to provide satisfactory drainage of this recurrent empyema.

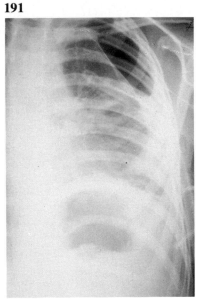

191 Air in the pleural space above an empyema indicates anaerobic infection which needs drainage.

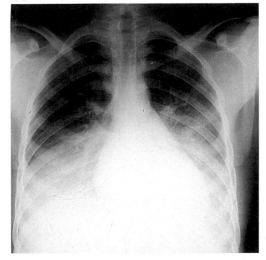

192 Bilateral lower lobe consolidation in an autosplenectomised sickle-cell disease patient. Lobar consolidation frequently develops in pneumococcal pneumonia although this extensive consolidation is unusual.

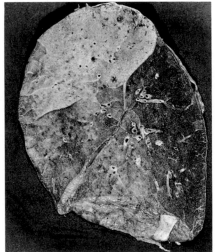

193 Pneumococcal pneumonia. Macroscopic section of whole lung in a fatal case of pneumococcal pneumonia of right upper lobe. The consolidation contrasts with the normal surrounding lung.

Klebsiella pneumonia

Klebsiella pneumonia is particularly seen in older males, alcoholics and in the malnourished. K. pneumoniae produces extensive haemorrhagic necrotising consolidation of the lung which may be fatal. There may be no significant leucocytosis.

194

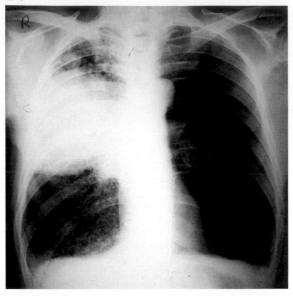

194 Pneumonic shadowing with bulging fissure developed in one week. Abscess effusion and empyema may occur.

195

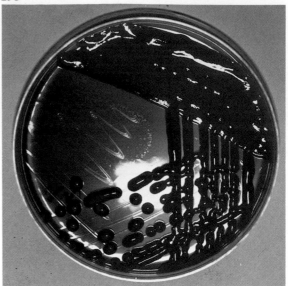

195 Klebsiella colonies on agar culture plate. Large mucoid coalescing colonies are present. The infected sputum is thick, red, gelatinous, like 'red-currant jelly' (MacConkey agar B reflected light).

Pneumonia in chronic lung disease
Pneumonia in chronic bronchitis and emphysema (COPD) is frequently caused by mixed infections with S. pneumoniae and H. influenzae.

196

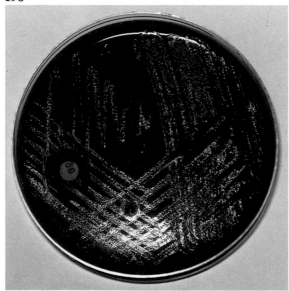

196 Sputum culture – mixed growth of H. influenzae and S. pneumoniae. The smaller H. influenzae colonies are inconspicuous against the larger S. pneumoniae colonies surrounded by their halo of α_1 haemolysis. (Blood agar reflected light.)

197

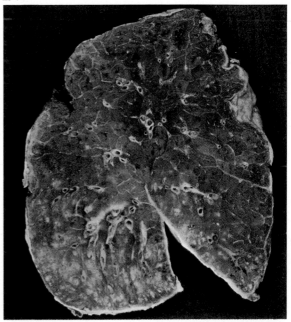

197 Bronchopneumonia with bronchiectasis in the left lower lobe and lingula of a bronchitic. Pale zones of consolidation, some relating to small bronchi, are present.

Staphylococcal pneumonia

Staphylococci cause less than 5 per cent of all bacterial pneumonias, except during influenza epidemics, but the disease is especially important because of its high mortality rate (up to 50 per cent).

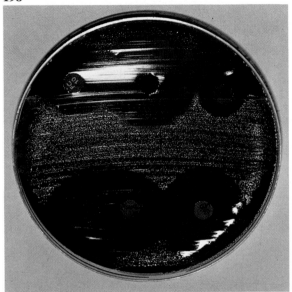

198 Staphylococcus aureus on blood agar culture. Note the inhibition of bacterial growth adjacent to the antibiotic impregnated discs.

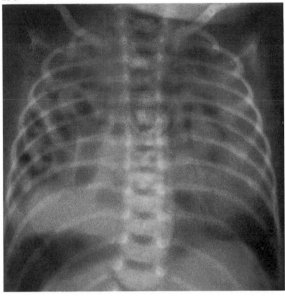

199 Primary staphylococcal pneumonia is more often seen in infants. Multiple pneumatoceles formed during the waning stage. Pneumothorax or pyopneumothorax results from rupture of a pneumatocele.

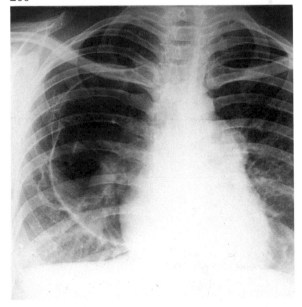

200 Large right lung pneumatocele after staphylococcal pneumonia. The large heart and pulmonary arteries are due to pulmonary hypertension which developed after repeated chest infections. A primary neutrophil disorder predisposed to infection. Pneumatoceles appear on the radiograph as air-filled, thin-walled cysts that change in size and appearance from day to day. Healing leads to radiographic resolution within a couple of weeks although rarely a stationary bulla-like shadow may remain.

Virus pneumonia

The most frequent pneumonia in epidemic form is caused by the influenza virus. Other true virus pneumonias are caused by parainfluenza, measles, varicella, respiratory syncytial virus, cytomegalovirus and adenoviruses.

In clinical practice, the differential diagnosis is from Q fever, psittacosis, mycoplasma pneumonia and Legionnaires' disease. These diseases cannot be distinguished on clinico-radiographic grounds, and precise diagnosis entails isolation of the organism and/or a four-fold rise in serum antibodies. Various new antiviral drugs act at different points in the adsorption and penetration of a virus into a cell, its intracellular synthesis, assembly and release (Figure **201**). Primary influenza virus infection causes tracheobronchitis and may progress to a haemorrhagic interstitial bronchopneumonia.

201

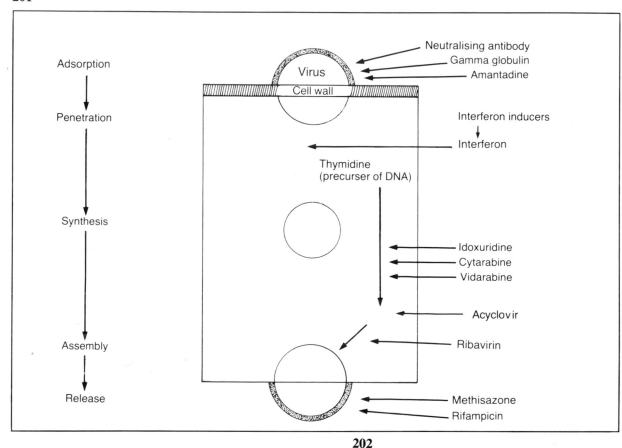

201 Chemical inhibition of viruses. A virus remains innocuous until it becomes intracellular. Various chemicals inhibit its growth at different metabolic stages of development.

202

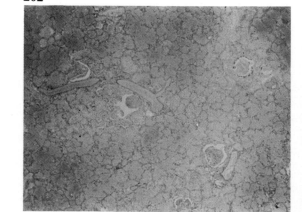

202 Primary influenza virus pneumonia. Massive haemorrhagic oedema fills the alveoli, and the respiratory epithelium is oedematous. During epidemics fit young adults may develop massive intra-alveolar haemorrhagic oedema and die of respiratory failure within 48 hours of onset of symptoms. In this instance no secondary bacterial infection was evident.

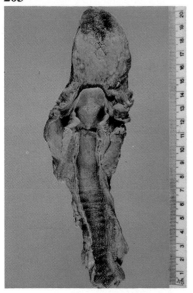

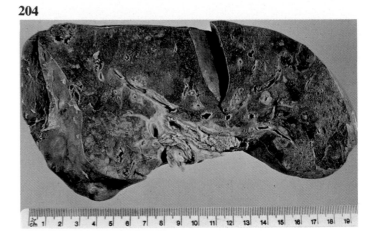

204 Combined influenza virus and bacterial pneumonia. Widespread consolidation and focal abscesses in this specimen are caused by staphylococcal pneumonia complicating influenza. Secondary bacterial pneumonia may be caused by S. pneumoniae, S. aureus, H. influenzae, S. pyogenes and P. aeruginosa.

203 Influenza tracheobronchitis. The brunt of the influenzal process affected the bronchial mucosa which is seen to be necrotic.

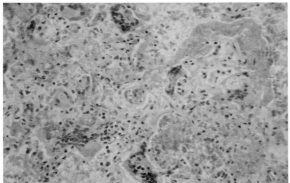

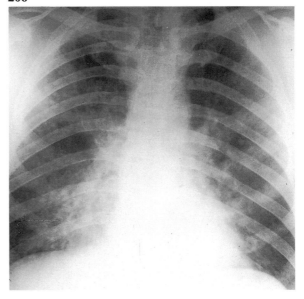

205 Measles virus pneumonia causes acute tracheobronchitis which may progress to an interstitial pneumonia with multinucleate giant cells, nuclear and cytoplasmic inclusion bodies. Fatal secondary bacterial bronchopneumonia is common in the malnourished and immunosuppressed.

Measles skin rash follows the prodromal symptoms by two to four days, and first appears behind the ears and on the face to spread downwards to the trunk and extremities. Discrete reddish brown macules may coalesce.

206 Pneumonia caused by chickenpox may complicate severe adult chickenpox. The xray shows diffuse nodular infiltration which may heal with miliary calcification (see **169**).

Chickenpox skin rash develops 10 to 23 days after exposure. Crops of umbilicated vesicles develop over the trunk and head.

Mycoplasma pneumoniae

Mycoplasma pneumoniae infections are endemic worldwide and responsible for localised outbreaks of pneumonia, tracheobronchitis, pharyngitis or myringitis. It is an acute penicillin-insensitive illness with a constitutional upset over-shadowing the respiratory symptoms at the onset. Fever usually lasts about one week and the radiographic changes persist for two to three weeks.

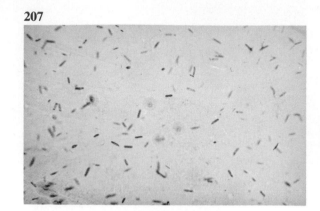

207 M. pneumoniae culture on agar. Mycoplasma may be isolated from sputum, which does not appear purulent as in bacterial pneumonia. The organism grows on blood agar. It lacks a rigid bacterial cell wall, so it is insensitive to the penicillins and cephalosporins. It is sensitive to tetracycline and erythromycin.

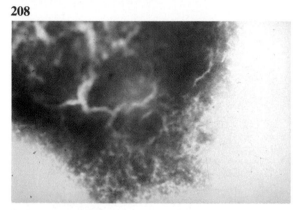

208 M. pneumoniae colony shown on glass cover slip imprint of blood agar culture. The single amorphous 'cotton wool' colony stains pink with Gram's stain.

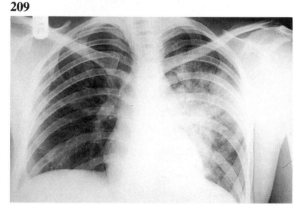

209 Consolidation and nodular opacities. There may be surprisingly few abnormal physical signs compared with widespread chest xray changes. The two dominant radiographic patterns are confluent areas of consolidation and nodular opacities. This radiograph was taken on the fifth day.

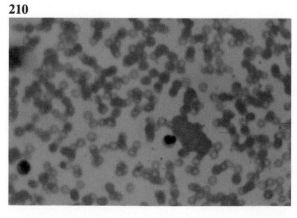

210 Cold agglutinins. Autoantibodies which agglutinate human red blood cells at 4°C will develop in the sera of 50 per cent of patients with M. pneumoniae infection during the second week of illness. The diagnosis is confirmed by isolation of the organism and raised mycoplasma complement-fixation test.

Legionnaires' disease

Legionnaires' disease is a form of severe pneumonia caused by an unusual aerobic Gram-negative bacillus, Legionella pneumophila. Outbreaks may be epidemic or sporadic.

The organism has been isolated from natural or polluted warm water and mud. Transmission of infection is presumed to be by inhalation of airborne organisms, especially from air conditioning plants cooling water.

The incubation period is from two to ten days. Respiratory symptoms are initially overshadowed by headache and confusion, muscle aches and mounting fevers. Asymptomatic infection may occur. Investigations may show a moderate leucocytosis with lymphopenia, hyponatraemia, abnormal liver function tests and haematuria. Histology shows a confluent bronchopneumonia and necrosis.

The demonstration of a four-fold rise in titre or an initial positive titre of greater than 1/256 of serum immunofluorescent antibody to the Legionnaires' bacillus is diagnostic. Death occurs in up to 20 per cent, the mortality being highest in the older age group and in the immunosuppressed.

211

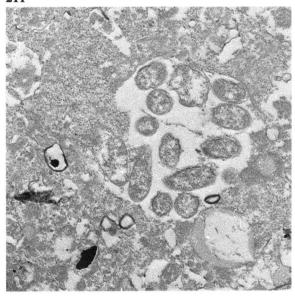

211 Legionella pneumophila organisms in lung tissue. The organisms are frequently intracellular and stain poorly if at all with Gram's stain. Complicated staining techniques are required if the organisms are to be reliably identified. *(EM ×10,000).*

Direct immunofluorescence is preferable; the test becomes positive during the second week of infection and IgM antibodies may persist for 18 months.

212a

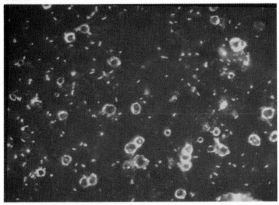

212a Legionella pneumophila. Smear of formalin-fixed lung tissue from a fatal case of Legionnaires' disease stained with FTIC – conjugated rabbit serum raised against Legionella pneumophila serogroup 1 stain. The organisms are shown by fluorescence.

212b

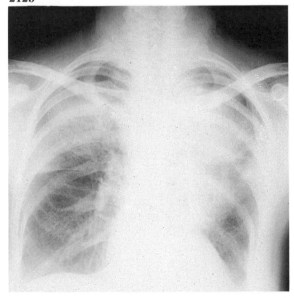

212b Extensive bilateral pneumonic shadowing with a small left pleural effusion. Legionnaires' disease should be considered in any patient with severe pneumonia which fails to respond to conventional antibiotic therapy.

Aspiration bronchopneumonia

Mucus and the resident oropharyngeal microbial flora are aspirated into one or more broncho-pulmonary segments causing collapse-consolidation of that segment. Most commonly affected are the right upper lobe and the apical segment of the lower lobes; these are the areas of the lung where inspired material is most likely to enter in the supine position.

Contributing factors include reduced levels of consciousness, alcoholism, anaesthetics, drugs; neurological or mechanical lesions of the upper gastro-intestinal tract; regurgitation from achalasia or an obstructive lesion of the oesophagus. The segments involved are delineated in Chapter 10.

The severity of the pneumonia depends upon the pathogenicity of the organisms inhaled and the efficacy of the local defences by broncho-pulmonary macrophages and the general resistance of the patients.

It is likely that bronchopneumonia is often caused by the spread of organisms from the upper to the lower respiratory tract.

Pneumonia after inhalation from the upper gastrointestinal tract is a far more serious event.

Massive inhalation of gastric contents may lead to sudden death from respiratory failure; inhalation of lesser amounts may lead to haemoptysis, haemorrhagic pneumonia and pulmonary oedema (acute adult respiratory distress syndrome).

213

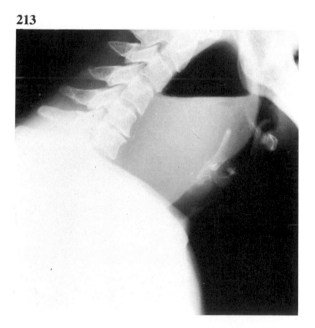

213 Secondary pneumonia caused by aspiration from this huge pharyngeal pouch.

214

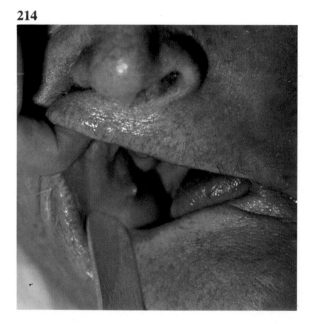

214 Bacterial parotitis. Elderly cachectic lady with terminal aspiration bronchopneumonia from bacterial parotitis.

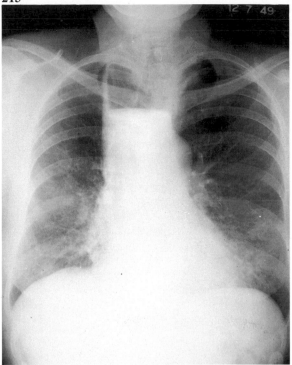

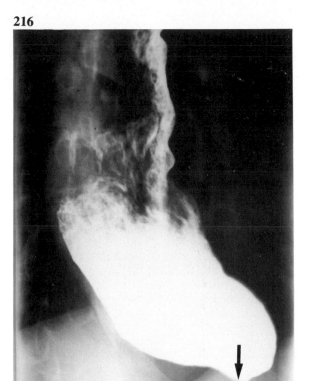

215 Achalasia of the oesophagus. Note the widened mediastinum, the fluid level in the upper oesophagus and the bilateral lower lobe shadowing caused by chronic overspill infection.

216 Oesophageal narrowing. The barium contrast study demonstrates terminal narrowing of the distended oesophagus (arrowed).

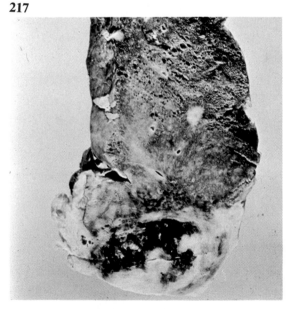

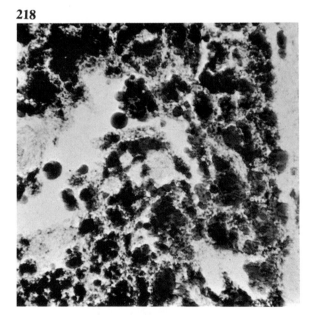

217 Lipoid 'paraffin' granuloma in the lower lobe developed as a result of the patient's long-standing ingestion of liquid paraffin in the mistaken hope of improving oesophageal achalasia. Similar lesions may follow aspiration of milk in infants, inhalation of oily nose drops, smoking black fat tobacco which contains oil, or unusually after intrabronchial injection of oil-based contrast medium for bronchography.

218 Pulmonary 'paraffin' granuloma. Microscopy shows diagnostic lipoid material stained red in biopsy specimen. *(Sudan IV ×100)*

15 Tuberculosis

Tuberculosis has a worldwide distribution. It is a common cause of morbidity or death in many developing countries and in some communities one per cent of the population have tubercle bacilli in their sputum.

In developed countries higher standards of nutrition and accommodation together with chemotherapeutic and other control measures practised during the past 30 years have helped to reduce both the mortality and overall prevalence of the disease. It remains high in some groups of patients – the diabetic, alcoholic, malnourished, those receiving corticosteroids or immunosuppressive drugs and in patients after gastrec-

tomy. In spite of the decline of tuberculosis in certain countries it still has numerous masquerades particularly in immigrants and in the ageing population.

Compared with an incidence of seven per 100,000 in Britain's native white population (**219**), the incidence is 200 per 100,000 in Britain's Asian immigrants rising to 500 per 100,000 in Asian males over 55 years of age.

In addition to this increased incidence, the Asian community also carries an increased resistance to streptomycin and isoniazid.

Mycobacterium tuberculosis and M. bovis are responsible for nearly all human infection.

219

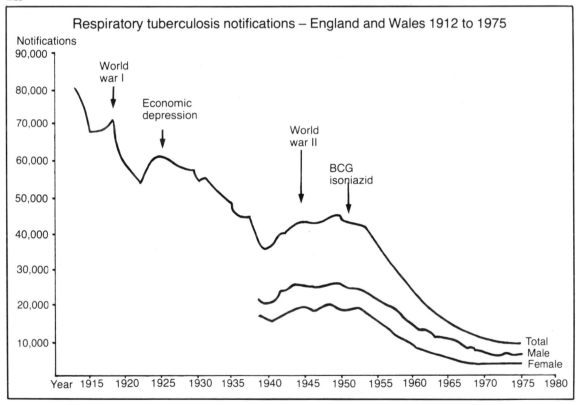

Respiratory tuberculosis notifications – England and Wales 1912 to 1975

Table: Masquerades of tuberculosis.

Myocardial disease
Peritonitis
Crohn's regional ileitis
Breast cancer
Sarcoidosis
Liver granulomas
Anonymous mycobacterial disease
Lymphadenopathy
Lymphocytic meningitis

Transmission of tubercle bacilli

Patients with active ulcerating pulmonary tuberculosis frequently expel an aerosol of tubercle bacilli suspended in droplets produced when speaking, sneezing or coughing, or in dust from dried sputum disseminated by clothes or handkerchiefs.

Droplets of about $1\,\mu m$ in diameter may penetrate directly to the alveoli and produce local infection.

Transmission by direct inoculation through the skin, cornea or buccal mucosa is rare. Mycobacterium bovis infection occurs through the alimentary canal from infected milk.

Diagnostic tests

220a

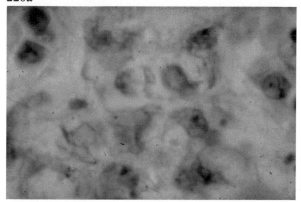

220b

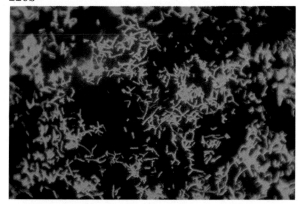

220a Direct sputum smear stained by Ziehl-Neelsen method. The rod-shaped bacteria do not stain readily, but once stained they resist decolourisation by alcohol or strong mineral acid solution. This quality of 'acid fastness' is a feature of the intact cell's waxy lipid-rich wall. If the direct smear is negative the centrifuged sputum sediment may be stained and examined. *(×1000)*

220b Fluorescent staining with auramine. Acid-fast bacilli appear as glowing fluorescent spots at low magnification. A large number of specimens may be rapidly examined using this technique. Culture is essential for diagnosis, for saprophytic non-pathogenic acid-fast bacilli will also be stained by auramine and Ziehl-Neelsen methods. *(×1000)*

221

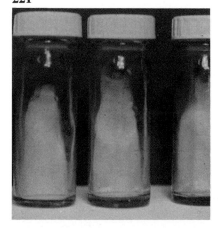

222

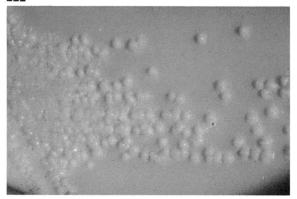

221 Mycobacterium tuberculosis culture on Löwenstein-Jensen medium slopes. Incubation of the inoculated medium at 37°C is continued for eight weeks. Mycobacterium tuberculosis is an obligate aerobe which grows best in an atmosphere enriched with 5 to 10 per cent carbon dioxide. It grows only at 37°C.

222 Mycobacterium tuberculosis culture. The slow-growing colonies are visible within three to four weeks, appearing cream-coloured, dry and wrinkled with irregular edges. Mycobacterium tuberculosis does not develop orange or yellow pigment in the presence of light and is positively identified by its ability to produce niacin. Isolated tubercle bacilli should be tested for drug susceptibility.

Atypical mycobacteria

Many acid-fast organisms may be confused with Mycobacterium tuberculosis; some are free-living saprophytes, some are associated with animals and some produce unequivocal disease closely resembling tuberculosis. These atypical mycobacteria are divided into groups according to pigmentation and growth rate (Table on page 91).

223

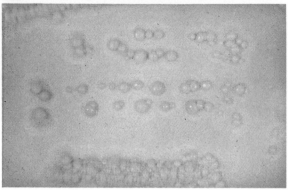

223 Mycobacterium kansasii are non-pigmented when grown in the dark but form rough yellow colonies in the light (photochromogen). Up to 60 per cent of atypical mycobacterial infections are caused by M. kansasii. It shows a predilection for older males, pneumoconiotic coal miners in France and Wales, and silicotic sandblasters in New Orleans.

224

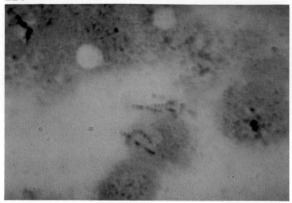

224 Mycobacterium kansasii. The direct smear shows acid-fast rods identical to those of Mycobacterium tuberculosis. (×1000)

225a

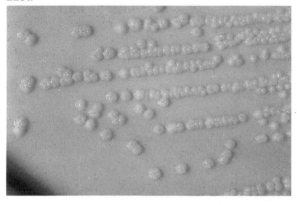

225a Mycobacterium fortuitum. White glistening colonies rapidly develop at 37°C (non-chromogen).

This rapidly growing mycobacterium may contaminate wounds or post-infection abscesses but is only rarely associated with lymphadenopathy or pulmonary disease.

225b

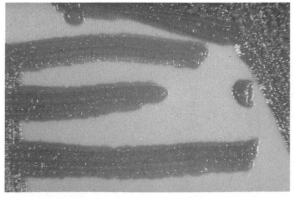

225b Mycobacterium scrofulaceum. Orange colonies grow in 10 to 14 days in the dark (scotochromogen).

226 Clinical examination of a patient with suspected tuberculosis.

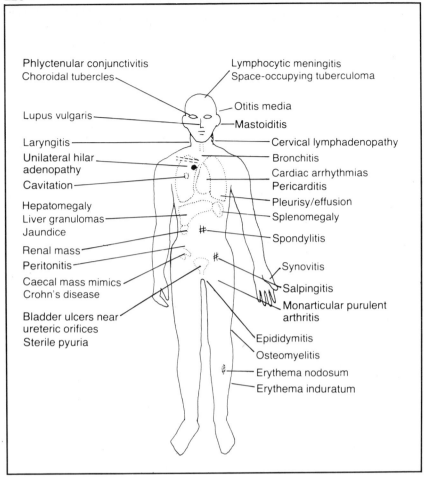

Phlyctenular conjunctivitis
Choroidal tubercles
Lymphocytic meningitis
Space-occupying tuberculoma
Lupus vulgaris
Otitis media
Mastoiditis
Laryngitis
Cervical lymphadenopathy
Unilateral hilar adenopathy
Bronchitis
Cardiac arrhythmias
Cavitation
Pericarditis
Pleurisy/effusion
Hepatomegaly
Liver granulomas
Splenomegaly
Jaundice
Spondylitis
Renal mass
Synovitis
Peritonitis
Salpingitis
Caecal mass mimics
Crohn's disease
Monarticular purulent arthritis
Bladder ulcers near ureteric orifices
Sterile pyuria
Epididymitis
Osteomyelitis
Erythema nodosum
Erythema induratum

Table: The opportunist mycobacteria.

Group	Mycobacterium species	Habitat and constitution	Human infection
Runyon I Photochromogen	M. kansasii	Water but not soil. Rarely isolated from animals. South to Central America, Europe	Pulmonary disease in middle-aged males with chronic underlying lung disease and poor defensive bronchopulmonary macrophages
Runyon II Scotochromogen	M. scrofulaceum	Soil and water worldwide	Lymphadenopathy Rarely lung disease
Runyon III Non-chromogen	M. xenopi (weak chromogen)	Water: river estuaries and coastal areas	Pulmonary disease and lymphadenopathy
	M. intracellulare (non-chromogenic)	Soil W. Australia and SE USA	
	M. avium (non-chromogenic)	Soil	
	M. fortuitum (non-chromogenic)	Soil Common contaminant	
Skin pathogens only	M. marinum M. balnei M. ulcerans (weak chromogens)	Water Swimming pools Fish tanks	Skin granulomas

Primary pulmonary tuberculosis

The primary lesion is subpleural. It may occur in any part of the lung although there is a bias towards the upper zones in adolescents and adults.

The regional lymph nodes draining the initial infection become involved; this combination is the primary complex or Ghon focus.

Uncomplicated primary tuberculosis seldom causes a significant illness and may pass unnoticed unless routine xray of the chest or tuberculin tests demonstrating conversion from negative to positive are carried out at the appropriate time.

Occasionally the infection progresses either locally in the lung or systemically with dissemination through the bloodstream. In young children tuberculous bronchopneumonia or life-threatening haematogenous miliary spread may occur. In adolescents and adults local extension with apical cavitation and fibrosis is more common.

227

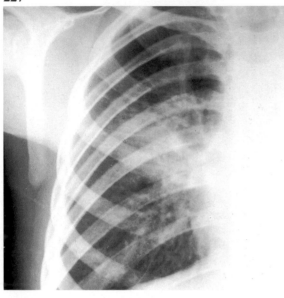

228

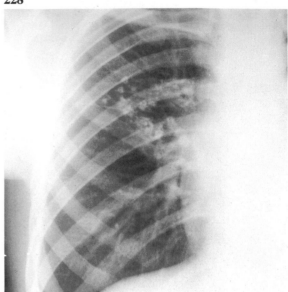

227 and 228   Primary infection in right upper lobe; healing with extensive calcification in the lung parenchyma.

229

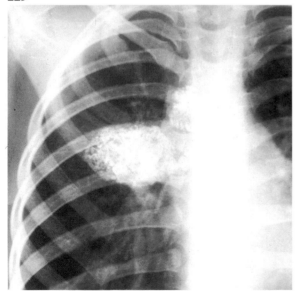

230

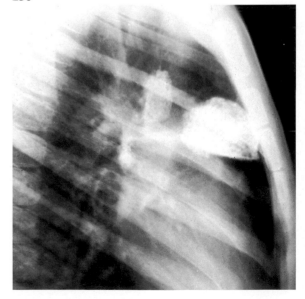

229 and 230   The healed primary complex with calcification in the lung and draining lymph node. This example shows an unusual amount of calcification in the healed tuberculoma and associated lymph node.

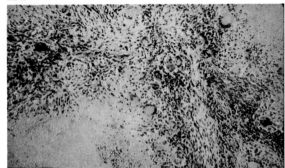

231 Tuberculous granuloma with caseation and giant cells. The neutrophils which characterise the initial inflammatory response are replaced by macrophages, and they eventually fuse into Langhans' giant cells and granulation tissue supervenes. Caseation is followed by healing with fibrosis. *(×60)*

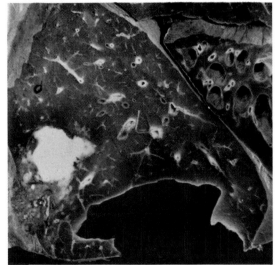

232 Peripheral Ghon focus in healed primary tuberculosis.

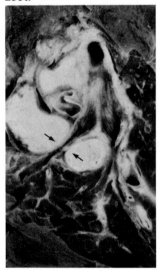

233a Tuberculous lymph nodes encircling and narrowing the right middle-lobe bronchus. Caseous material discharged from the nodes into the bronchial lumen resulted in widespread tuberculous pneumonia.

233b and c 'Middle lobe' syndrome. The bronchogram demonstrates bronchiectasis in the middle lobe, which is also shown in the resected right middle lobe surgical specimen. The enlarged tuberculous lymph nodes, present in the glass specimen tube (arrowed), compressed the right middle-lobe bronchus causing distal collapse and infection. This commonly affects the middle-lobe bronchus because it is encircled by lymphatic tissue.

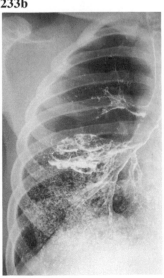

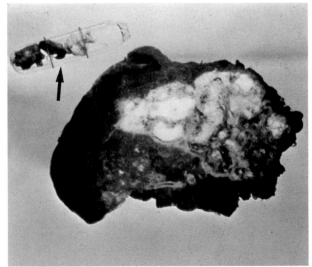

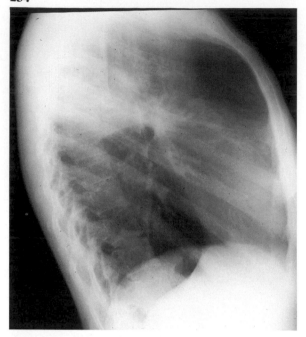

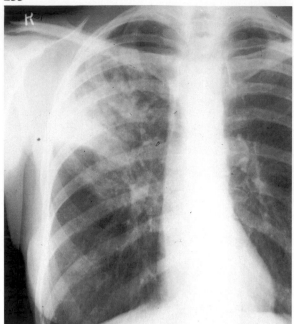

234 and 235 Tuberculous pneumonia resembling an acute bacterial pneumonia is seen when the alveoli are flooded with bacilli from an area of liquid necrosis. The patient presented with rigors, fever, pleuritic chest pain and a productive cough. The radiographic clue to the diagnosis of tuberculosis is the involvement of the posterior and apical segments of the upper lobe.

236

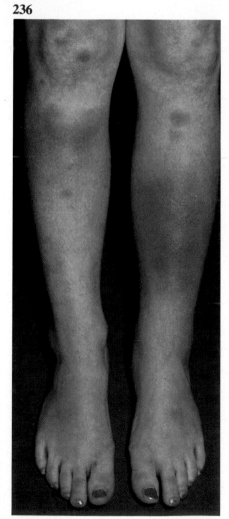

236 Erythema nodosum is a manifestation of the presence of circulating immune complexes. It may infrequently accompany primary tuberculosis within a few weeks of tuberculin conversion. Pain in the joints may occur with swelling mimicking rheumatic fever. Erythema nodosum is a non-specific hypersensitivity phenomenon. It is particularly common in women of childbearing age. There are numerous causes of this physical sign (see table on page 95).

Table: Conditions associated with erythema nodosum.

Associated disease	Age	Clinical features	Xray	Skin test	Laboratory confirmation
Sarcoidosis	20 to 40 Rare below 20 or over 50	Female preponderance Lymphadenopathy uveitis or conjunctivitis	Bilateral hilar adenopathy ± pulmonary infiltration	Kveim-Siltzbach test positive Tuberculin test negative	Histology of inflamed scar tissue Hypercalcaemia Serum angiotensin-converting enzyme
Streptococcal infection	Any	Preceding upper respiratory tract infection	—	—	ß-haemolytic strepto-coccus in throat Raised anti-streptolysin titre
Tuberculosis	Under 20	Asian migrant close contact with tuberculosis Primary complex	Unilateral hilar adenopathy Ghon focus	Tuberculin conver-sion to high degree of positivity	Isolation of Mycobacterium tuberculosis
Drugs	Any	Transfer factor Sulphonamides Oral contraceptives Sulphones, penicillin Levamisole	—	—	Recurs when rechallenged with drug
Histoplasmosis	Any	From Ohio Respiratory symptoms Lymphadenopathy	Miliary mottling	Histoplasmin	Complement-fixation test Fungal hyphae in sputum or lung biopsy
Coccidioido-mycosis	Any	From California Respiratory symptoms Flu-like illness	Miliary mottling Hilar glands or cavitation	Coccidioidin	Complement-fixation test Fungus in sputum or lung biopsy
Leprosy (lepromatous)	Any	From 'tropics' Symmetrical nodular rash Iridocyclitis Patchy sensory loss	Normal	Lepromin	Isolate M. leprae: skin or nerve biopsy
Ulcerative colitis	15 to 40	Diarrhoea	Ba. enema	—	Rectal biopsy
Crohn's disease	15 to 40	Abdominal pain, fever, fistulae	Ba. follow-through, Ba. enema	Depression of delayed-type hypersensitivity	Intestinal biopsy
Yersinia infection	Any	Particularly France and Scandinavia Abdominal pain, diarrhoea	Normal chest xray and barium studies	—	Stool culture: Y. enterocolitica Raised agglutinin titres
Pregnancy	15 to 40	First trimester	—	—	Recurs with next pregnancy
Circulating immune complex	Any	Polyarthralgia Uveitis Meningism	—	—	High ESR Positive tests by various techniques Raji, Ciq, etc.

237

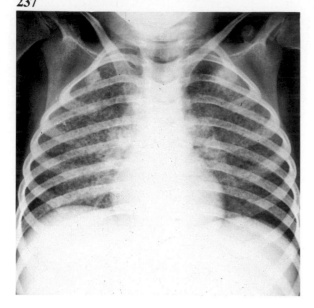

Miliary tuberculosis results from the rupture of a caseating primary focus or from a caseating lesion in the intima of a blood vessel that discharge bacilli throughout the bloodstream.

237   Acute and fatal miliary tuberculosis in a six-year-old child. The right paratracheal lymph gland is enlarged and miliary shadows are present in both lung fields. Miliary tuberculosis implies blood-borne dissemination.

238   Miliary tuberculosis. Numerous caseating pulmonary granulomas.

239   Choroidal tubercles in acute miliary tuberculosis. Their presence is pathognomonic. In adult chronic miliary tuberculosis choroidal tubercles are rarely present.

240   Tuberculous meningitis. The meninges are studded with small tubercles and the base of the brain covered by a fibrinous exudate. Miliary spread to the brain is most common in childhood and occurs within the first year of infection. This classic case presented with fever, hepatosplenomegaly and choroidal tubercles.

241   Miliary tuberculosis. Hepatic involvement with caseating granulomas. In difficult cases liver biopsy may be helpful.

238

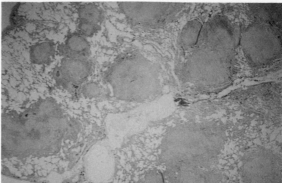

239

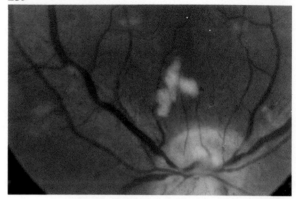

240

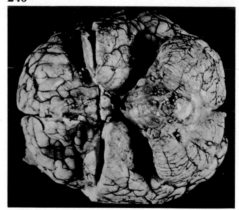

241

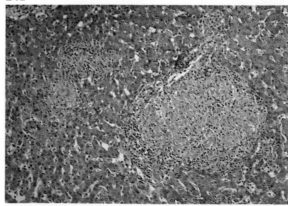

Compliciations of primary tuberculosis

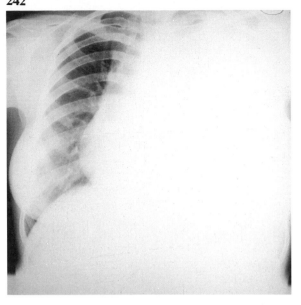

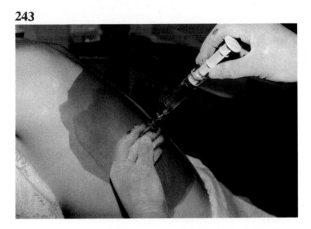

243   Therapeutic aspiration of a tuberculous effusion. Pleural biopsy is done at the same time. It may be diagnostic in tuberculosis and pleural carcinomatosis. Note the characteristic straw-coloured fluid in the syringe. The protein content was 43 g/litre and lymphocytes were present in large numbers.

242   Tuberculous pleural effusion presenting with a three-month history of pleural pain, malaise, drenching sweats and progressive dyspnoea. This massive effusion fills the left pleural cavity and displaces the mediastinum to the right. Tuberculous effusions tend to form three to six months after the primary infection.

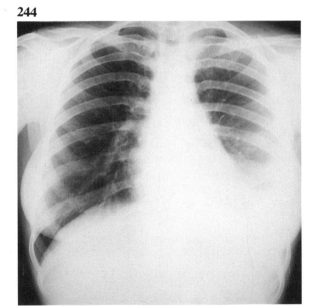

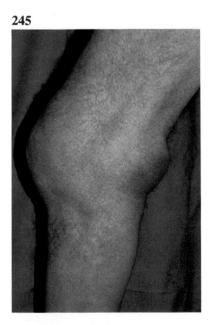

244   Tuberculous pleural effusion after aspiration of 5 litres of fluid. Note the central position of the mediastinum. (Same patient as **242**.)

245   Tuberculous effusion of the knee with marked wasting of the quadriceps. This alcoholic male failed to attend for treatment of pulmonary tuberculosis three years before presenting with a painful swollen knee. The knee joint was destroyed and arthrodesis required.

246

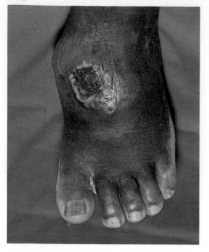

246 Tuberculous osteomyelitis presenting with a deep ulcer in foot. Bone involvement usually occurs within three years of the primary infection.

247

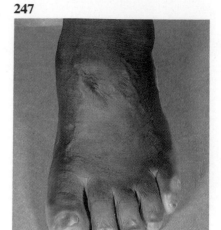

247 Tuberculous osteomyelitis. After anti-tuberculous chemotherapy, the ulcer healed.

248

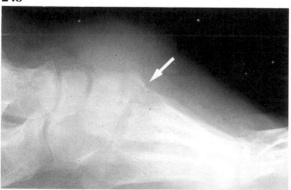

248 Tuberculous osteomyelitis with bone destruction (arrowed). Note the soft tissue swelling. (Same patient as **246**.)

249

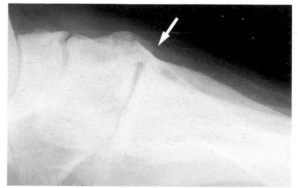

249 Tuberculous osteomyelitis. Eventual healing by bony fusion (arrowed). (Same patient as **247**.)

250

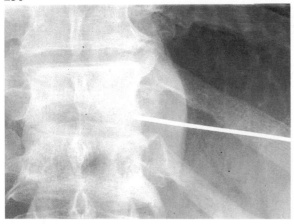

250 Tuberculous paravertebral abscess (Pott's disease) involving the lumbar vertebrae in an adult. The needle lies in the abscess cavity. Narrowing of the disc space is soon followed by destruction of adjacent vertebral bodies. This patient experienced troublesome back pain for two years before the correct diagnosis was made. The hip, spine and weight-bearing joints are most commonly affected by skeletal tuberculosis.

251

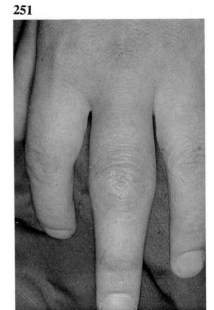

251 Tuberculous dactylitis commonly involves the metaphysis.

252

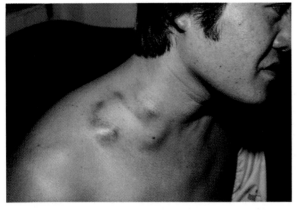

252 Tuberculous involvement of cervical lymph nodes (scrofula). Glandular tuberculosis is now rare in Europeans, but still common in Asians.

253

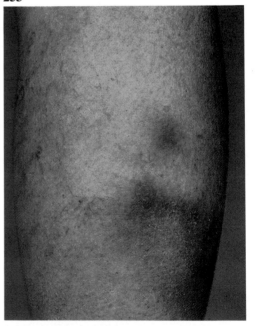

253 Erythema induratum (Bazin's disease). Symmetrical chilblain-like lesions develop on the calves of young women. The attack usually begins in cold weather. The lesions may ulcerate.

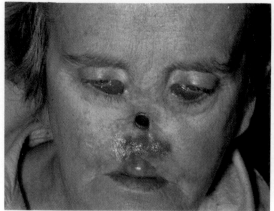
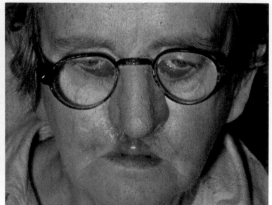

254a Lupus vulgaris begins with ulceration of the nasolabial fold. Gradual extension of this tuberculous inflammation leads to complete destruction of the nose. This patient was fitted with an artificial nose (**254b**) which proved to be a cosmetic success.

Postprimary pulmonary tuberculosis

This is numerically the most common and important type of tuberculosis, for the infected sputum is the main source of continuing disease in the community.

The earliest lesions are aggregations of tubercles with collapse and consolidation of alveoli. These lesions may remain localised and confined by fibrosis, representing a compromise between destruction and repair. Caseation may occur. Cavities form if the caseous pus is discharged into a bronchus. Small vessels may thrombose or erode.

Many tuberculous patients remain asymptomatic; their disease is only recognised by routine chest xray.

Cavitation may be accompanied by weightloss, productive cough, purulent sputum, haemoptysis and fever.

Postprimary tuberculosis may follow:
1 Progression of a primary lesion. In Europe and North America the primary infection often occurs in adolescence or adult life.
2 Reactivation of a primary lesion. The poor cellular immunity which occurs with drugs or old age may lead on to reactivation of a dormant primary complex.
3 Exogenous superinfection. Most patients with a healed primary complex mount a successful immune reaction when re-exposed to tuberculosis. Superinfection may overwhelm these defences.

255

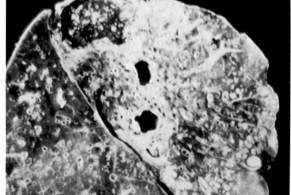

255 Postprimary tuberculosis with healing cavity.

256

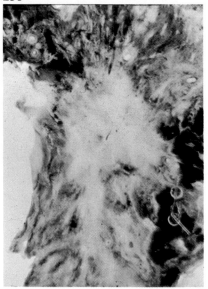

256 Postprimary tuberculosis. The cavity has healed and dense fibrous tissue has formed.

257

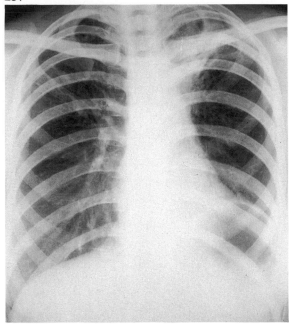

257 Upper lobe consolidation and an apical cavity. Sputum was heavily infected with acid-fast bacilli.

258

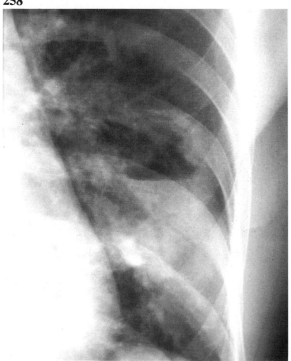

258 Cavitating tuberculosis. A fluid-filled cavity lies in the left lower lobe; the sputum was positive. In cavitating tuberculosis large numbers of organisms are expectorated. Diagnosis should be readily made by examining the sputum.

259

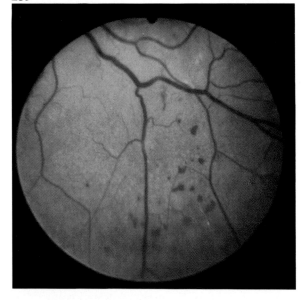

259 Diabetic retinopathy. Microaneurysms and exudates in the retina. There is an increased incidence of tuberculosis among diabetic patients. The possibility of diabetes should be considered in all patients with tuberculosis.

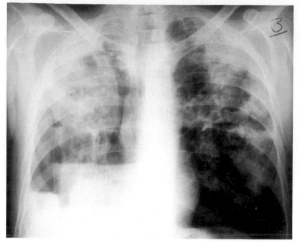

260 **Secondary pneumothorax** with loculated haemorrhagic effusion and widespread bronchopneumonic shadowing. The healed rib fractures are a common finding in the alcoholic. The alcoholic cirrhotic malnourished vagrant is prone to reactivation of tuberculosis and to discontinuing therapy before cure is effected. The serum total bilirubin concentration was elevated.

261 **Micronodular cirrhosis.** Many of the hepatocytes are necrotic and there is a marked fatty infiltration. The biopsy was taken from a patient with alcoholic cirrhosis and tuberculosis. Hepatotoxic antituberculous drugs should be given under close supervision with serial measurement of liver function. Most cirrhotic patients tolerate antituberculous drugs well; their liver function improves with abstinence from alcohol and with an adequate intake of protein.

262 **Tuberculous 'collar stud' abscess** from cervical lymph nodes pointing in the neck. Cervical node enlargement is a particularly common extrapulmonary manifestation in Asian immigrants caused by secondary rather than 'primary complex' tuberculosis. Evidence of tuberculosis may not be found elsewhere.

263 **Tuberculous abscess.** A ragged chronic discharging sinus developed. The tuberculous glands often lie beneath the deep fascia and discharge caseous pus. Diagnosis is best established by gland biopsy; culture of the lymph node or pus is less successful. Surgical drainage with curettage and routine antituberculous therapy is curative.

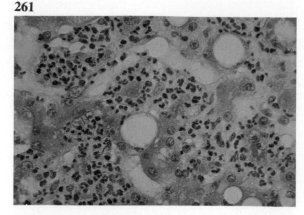

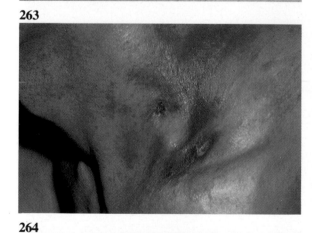

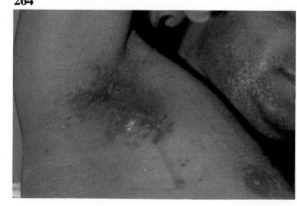

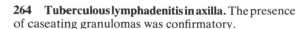

264 **Tuberculous lymphadenitis in axilla.** The presence of caseating granulomas was confirmatory.

265

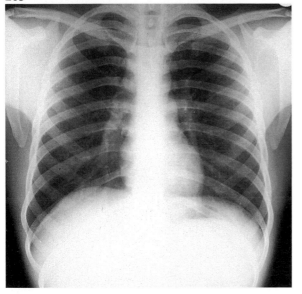

265 Right paratracheal gland enlargement. The direct sputum smear was positive for acid-fast bacilli.

266

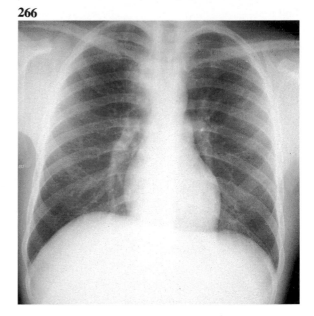

266 Right paratracheal gland enlargement. Same patient as **265** after 140 days' supervised chemotherapy. Lymph glands may enlarge and caseate during adequate treatment.

267

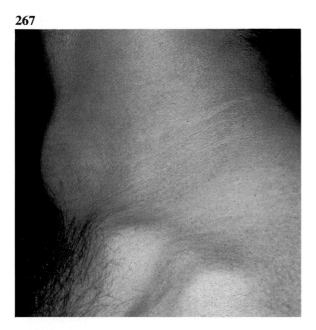

267 Right paratracheal gland enlargement. Same patient as **265**. A fluctuant swelling appeared at the sternal notch from which 60 ml of sterile caseous material was aspirated.

Prolonged chemotherapy and curettage were necessary to settle this patient's disease.

268

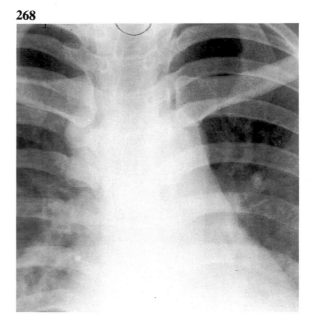

268 Tuberculous right paratracheal lymphadenopathy. This immigrant patient presented with night sweats, malaise, weightloss and a strongly positive tuberculin test. Routine 'first line' antituberculous treatment was begun.

269

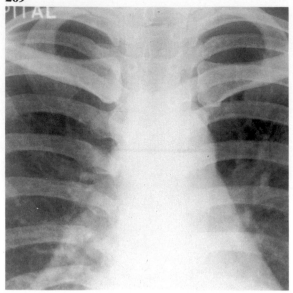

270

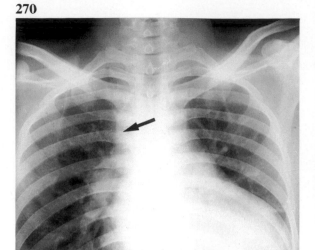

269 Tuberculous right paratracheal lymphadeno-pathy. The clinical response to eight weeks' drug treatment was satisfactory. The xray shows shrinkage of the previously enlarged nodes (same patient as **268**).

270 Tuberculous pericardial effusion. The cardiac silhouette is widened and has a globular shape. Culture of the aspirated fluid grew tubercle bacilli. One clue to the diagnosis was the enlarged right paratracheal lymph gland (arrowed).

271

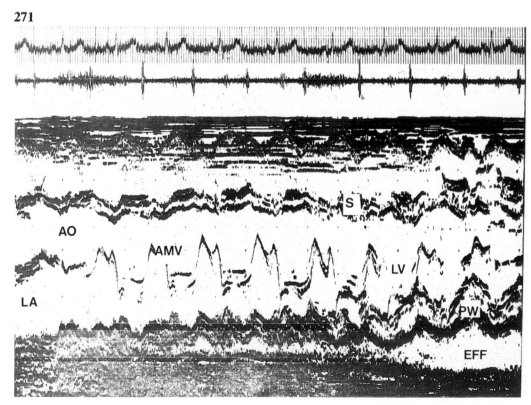

271 M. Mode Echo scan of the heart showing a large posterior pericardial effusion.

LA = left atrium
AO = aorta
AMV = anterior leaflet of mitral valve

S   = septum
LV = left ventricular cavity
PW = posterior cardiac wall
EFF = pericardial effusion

272

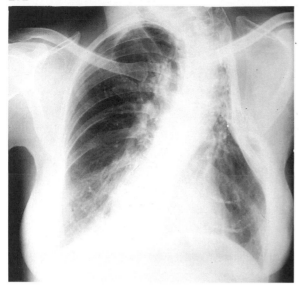

272 Thoracoplasty performed to collapse the left upper lobe cavity; 25 years later the lateral spine curvature has increased and there is calcification in the collapsed portion of lung, but the patient is otherwise well.

273

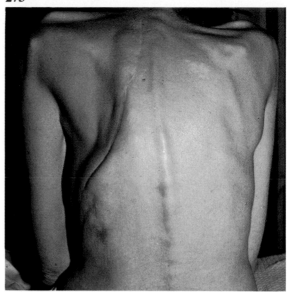

273 Deformity resulting from thoracoplasty.

Pulmonary complications as a sequel to healed tuberculosis

274

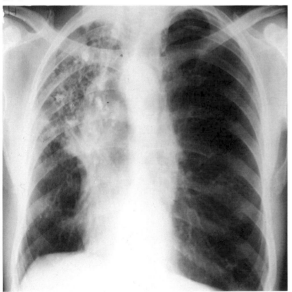

274 Extensive fibrosis of right upper lobe with calcification as a sign of old pulmonary tuberculosis. The mediastinum is deviated to the right.

275

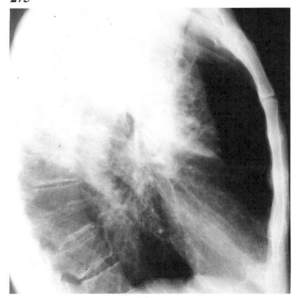

275 Extensive fibrosis of right upper lobe. The lateral film shows a large anterior window caused by the left lung herniating across to the right. (Same patient as **274**.)

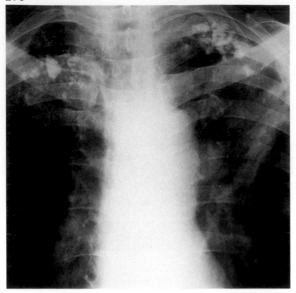

276 Extensive bilateral apical calcification from healed tuberculosis. Modern antituberculous chemotherapy combined with public health measures should reduce the numbers of patients whose lungs are extensively damaged by tuberculosis.

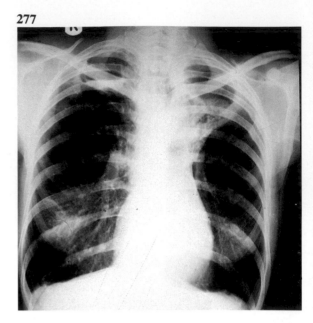

277 Pulmonary tuberculosis with bilateral apical calcification which healed with chemotherapy.

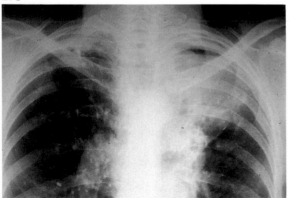

278 Aspergilloma. Fourteen years later a huge aspergilloma has developed. A translucent halo of air surrounds a dense circular opacity. Aspergilloma develops in 20 per cent of open healed tuberculous cavities and may cause severe haemoptysis.

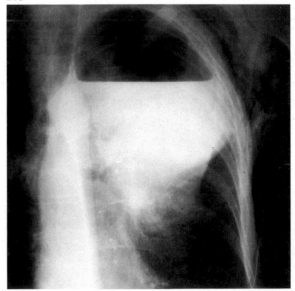

279 Aspergilloma. Sixteen years later the cavity has become secondarily infected. The fluid level is a sign that drainage of fluid is occurring.

Skin tests for tuberculosis

Cell-mediated delayed hypersensitivity to tuberculin protein develops four to eight weeks after infection with tubercle bacilli and is demonstrated by intradermal injections of a purified protein derivative of tuberculin (PPD) or heat concentrated tuberculin (HCSM). The potency of PPD is expressed in terms of international units (IU) per ml.

Standard Mantoux test dilutions (UK)

Labelled dilution on container	Labelled potency on container	Potency of 0.1 ml dose injected
1/10000	10 IU per ml	1 IU
1/1000	100 IU per ml	10 IU
1/100	1000 IU per ml	100 IU

280

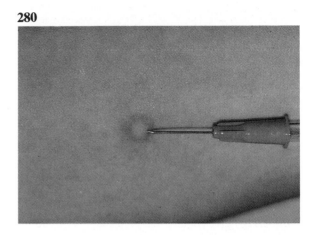

280 Mantoux skin test. 0.1 ml of a standard dilution of PPD prepared from M. tuberculosis is injected intradermally using a tuberculin syringe and intradermal needle (25G 16mm long with short bevel). Routine testing in the UK is done with PPD 10 IU while PPD 5 IU is used for the standard test in the USA. PPD is available prepared from atypical and avian mycobacteria.

281

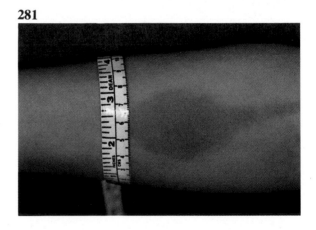

281 Mantoux 10 IU positive reaction at 48 hours. 30mm induration and with vesiculation in a strongly hypersensitive subject. The Mantoux skin test is read between 48 and 72 hours. The UK recommendations imply that the widest diameter of induration is measured; induration of 6mm or greater indicates a positive reaction. In the USA it is recommended that the diameter of induration is measured in millimetres transversely to the long axis of the forearm; 5mm to 9mm induration is regarded as a doubtful positive and 10mm induration or greater as positive. A doubtful positive is equated with the alternative possibility of non-specific atypical mycobacterial infection. Induration seldom occurs without a surrounding halo of erythema; this erythema is ignored when measuring the response.

282

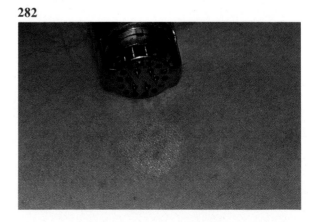

282 The Heaf multiple tuberculin test. This simple instrument has six spring-loaded needles which introduce undiluted tuberculin (PPD 100 000 IU per ml) into the skin. The depth of penetration can be adjusted; 1 mm is recommended for infants and 2 mm for older children and adults. A drop of PPD is applied to the cleansed dry skin of the forearm. The instrument is applied at right angles to the skin and the end plate firmly pressed on the centre of the film of tuberculin. The release of the mechanism allows the needles to pierce the skin and carry with them some tuberculin. The test, which is at least as strong as a Mantoux 10 IU test, is read at 48 to 96 hours. There are four well-defined grades of reaction.

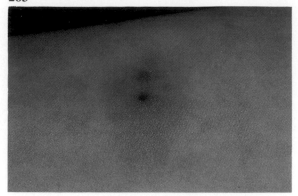

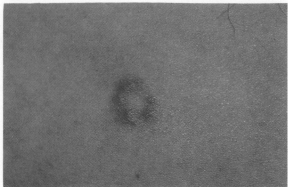

283

284

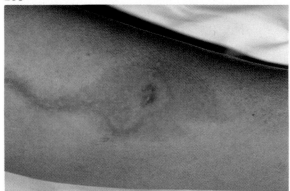

285

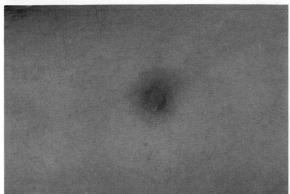

286

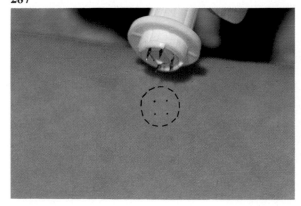

287

283 Heaf test – grade 1. Discrete palpable induration at four or more of the puncture points.

284 Heaf test – grade 2. The papules are larger and have coalesced to form a ring.

285 Heaf test – grade 3. More intensive induration. The papules are larger still and have formed a solid central plaque.

286 Heaf test – grade 4. Extensive induration and surrounding erythema. The plaque is surmounted by vesicles which have fused resulting in early central ulceration. This is a severe reaction with lymphangitis and regional lymphadenitis which caused fever and malaise.

When tuberculosis is suspected Mantoux PPD 1 IU should be used as a first test to prevent unnecessarily severe reaction.

287 The tuberculin tine test is a disposable multi-puncture test comparable to a Mantoux 5 IU PPD test. The four tines, coated with highly purified undiluted old tuberculin (OT), are firmly pressed on the skin of the forearm for two seconds. Palpable induration is measured after 48 to 72 hours.

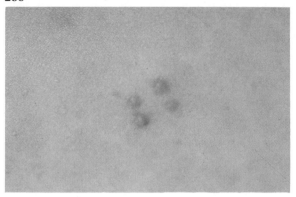

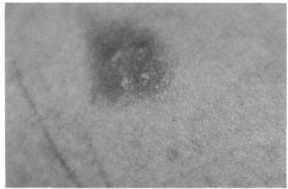

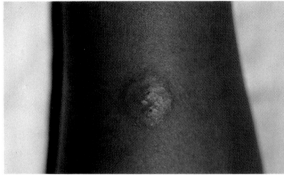

288 Tine test – negative reaction. The diameter of induration of the largest single reaction is measured. The official recommendations are that induration of 2 mm or less is recorded as a negative reaction. The results of the tine test are similar to the Heaf test and some authorities suggest an identical grading system. This example shows discrete palpable induration at the four puncture sites, and would be comparable to a grade 1 Heaf test.

289 Tine test – doubtful positive reaction. The size of induration of the largest single reaction is from 2 mm to 4 mm. The papules are touching but leaving a central depression which would be comparable to a grade 2 Heaf reaction.

290 Tine test – positive reaction. 5 mm or more induration is a positive reaction. The plaque is surmounted by vesicles at the original puncture points and surrounded by erythema. This reaction would be comparable to a grade 4 Heaf test.

BCG vaccination

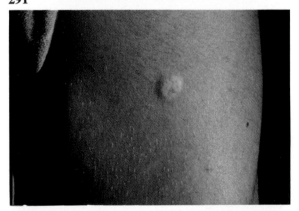

291 Intradermal immunisation using BCG vaccination (Bacille Calmette-Guérin, an attenuated bovine mycobacteria). A cutaneous primary complex forms at the vaccination site. Vaccination is contraindicated if there is hypogammaglobulinaemia, in atopic patients with eczema, and in patients with tuberculosis or a positive tuberculin skin test. It is estimated that BCG confers an 80 per cent protection against tuberculosis which lasts for about 15 years.

In developing countries BCG vaccination can provide a cheap and effective method of reducing the incidence of tuberculosis. Vaccination within the previous three weeks to smallpox, polio or yellow fever is a relative contraindication to BCG vaccination.

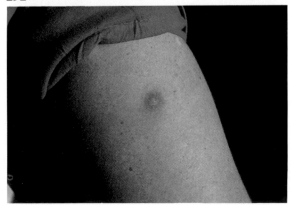

292 BCG second to fourth week. Indurated papule which becomes scaly.

293

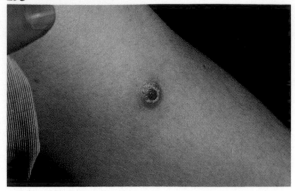

293 BCG sixth week. Crusting and a dry scab forms.

294

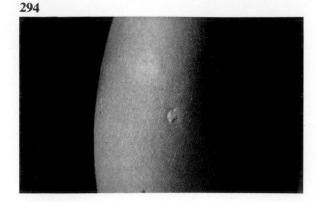

294 BCG scar. The ulcer heals leaving a depressed white scar.

295

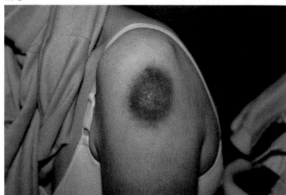

295 BCG abscess. This abscess developed at the site of BCG injection two years after vaccination, and BCG organisms were isolated from the pus.

296a

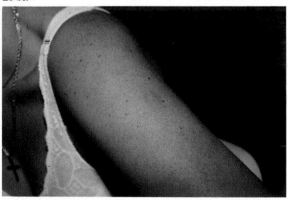

296a BCG abscess at the site of vaccination which caused pain 18 months after injection. Pus was aspirated and BCG organisms were identified.

296b

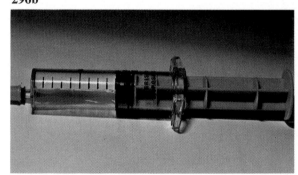

296b BCG pus aspirated from arm of patient shown in 296a.

16 Other infections

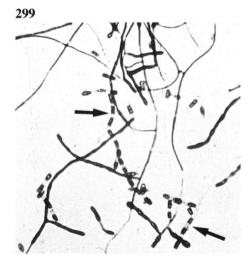

Coccidioidomycosis

Coccidioidomycosis is a fungus infection acquired in the arid regions of the Southern USA and Latin America. A respiratory infection follows the inhalation of spores. In some patients the only evidence of the infection is the development of precipitating antibodies and positive skin tests, while others will develop an influenza-like illness with fever, malaise, cough and arthralgia. Hypersensitivity reactions with erythema nodosum may develop in 5 to 10 per cent of infected individuals.

Coccidioides immitis is dimorphic, existing in living tissue as spherules and as a mycelial form in soil and on routine culture.

Although most infections are mild, C. immitis may cause a fatal widely disseminated disease, especially in the immunocompromised.

Synonyms include San Joaquin fever, valley fever or desert rheumatism.

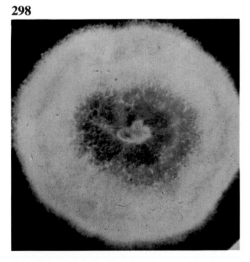

298 Coccidioides immitis grows on culture as white to tan fluffy mycelium composed of septate hyphae. The culture has no specific characteristics and therefore identification is made by demonstrating spherules in the tissues of an infected host.

299 Hyphae form alternating arthrospores and empty cells (arrowed). The arthrospores are light and, if inhaled, are highly infectious, developing into tissue spherules. They are produced on specialised lateral branches of the vegetative hyphae. The fertile part of these branches expands and septation occurs. Alternate cells grow larger and develop into arthrospores, while cells between the spores lose cytoplasm.

Arthrospores have the ability to change into spherules in host tissue and also in special culture conditions.

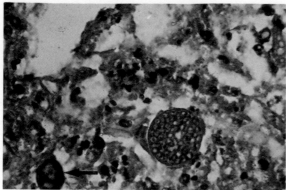

300 A mature spherule with endospores. Tissue from a lung biopsy. Spherules vary from 20 to 100 μm in diameter and only develop in animal hosts. When mature, up to 10^5 endospores may be released. An immature spherule is also shown (arrowed). It has a clear centre with peripheral cytoplasm and a prominent thick wall. *(H&E ×100)*

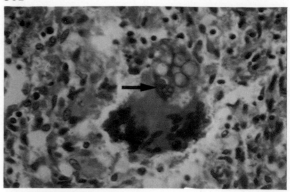

301 Granuloma with spherules. A lung biopsy from a patient with pulmonary coccidioidomycosis. This spherule has ruptured (arrowed) and only a small portion of the wall remains. The spherules lie adjacent to a Langhans' giant cell. *(H&E ×200)*

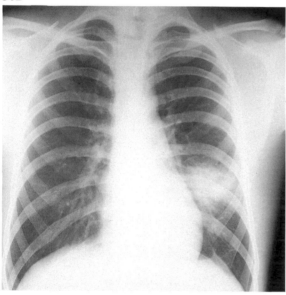

302 Chronic coccidioidomycosis. This coin lesion was a coccidioidoma. The diagnosis was made by aspiration needle biopsy.

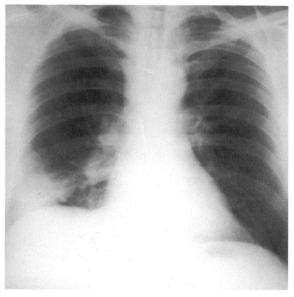

303 Acute coccidioidomycosis with hilar and paratracheal lymphadenopathy and right basal pneumonia. Effusions may also occur.

Skin test. Delayed hypersensitivity to intradermal injection of coccidioidin (a filtrate of broth culture of C. immitis) or spherulin (a sterile filtrate from culture spherules) develops three days to three weeks after the onset of symptoms. Maximum induration is reached 24 to 48 hours after injection. IgM precipitins are detectable in 90 per cent of patients within four weeks of infection and are followed by complement-fixing IgG antibodies. The persistence of precipitins or increasing titres of complement-fixing antibodies is associated with dissemination and a poor prognosis.

Actinomycosis

Actinomycosis is a chronic suppurative infection caused by Actinomyces israelii and related to anaerobic filamentous bacteria. These organisms are normal saprophytes which are present in the oral cavity. Cervico-facial infections are most common, but rarely the lungs or abdomen may be affected.

304

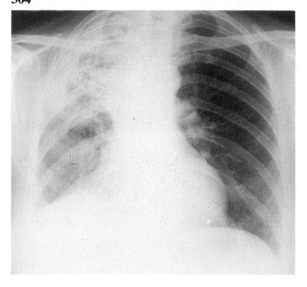

304 Pulmonary actinomycosis may follow aspiration of saliva into the lung. A low-grade pneumonitis develops with fever and a productive cough, followed by spread to the pleura resulting in empyema and sinuses of the chest wall.

305

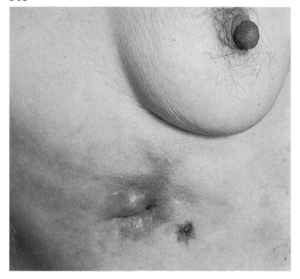

305 Multiple draining sinuses. Untreated actinomycosis will lead to chronic persistent infection. Periosteal reactions may result in new bone formation on the undersurface of the ribs. Surgical drainage of the infection and prolonged intravenous administration of penicillin with probenecid are effective.

306

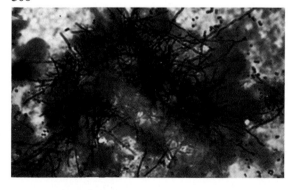

306 Actinomycosis. 'Sulphur' granules are diagnostic and consist of colonies of Gram-positive mycelial filaments surrounded by eosinophilic 'clubs'. The mycelial filaments often show irregular staining which gives a beaded appearance. The eosinophilic 'clubs' may be antigen-antibody complexes and probably indicate host resistance.

307

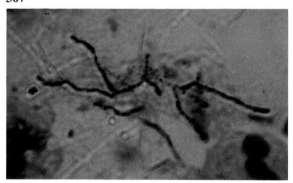

307 Actinomycosis. Gram-positive branching mycelial filaments and pus cells in sputum. *(Gram-stain ×960)*

113

308 **A colony of actinomyces in the lung.** In the centre is a dense mass of mycelial filaments. The periphery of radially arranged eosinophilic 'clubs' is surrounded by polymorphonuclear leucocytes. *(H&E ×350)*

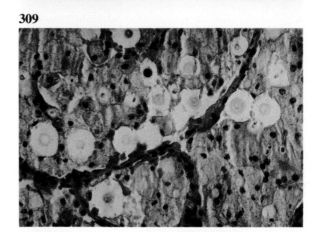

308

Cryptococcosis

Cryptococcus neoformans is a yeast occurring widely in nature, particularly in bird droppings. Massive infection may result in progressive systemic disease in the otherwise healthy, but most infections occur in the immunodeficient or immunosuppressed (page 123). Pulmonary disease is the commonest presentation, for the lung is the principal site of entry of fungus.

309 **Cryptococcus neoformans in lung showing capsules.** *(Alcian blue and haematoxylin ×100)*

309

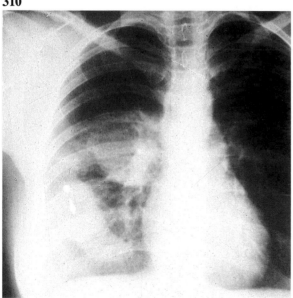

310

310 **Cryptococcus neoformans infiltration of right lower and middle lobe.**

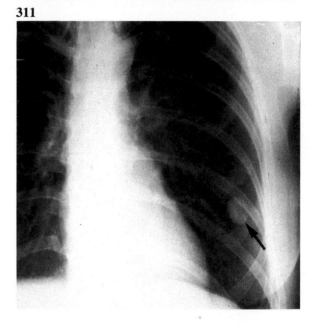

311

311 **Subpleural coin lesion.** Pulmonary cryptococcosis is usually transient and not severe. No radiographic features are characteristic but diffuse infiltration of the lower lobes is common while hilar adenopathy, coin lesions, collapse and effusions are rare. Histology of wedge resection gave the diagnosis.

312

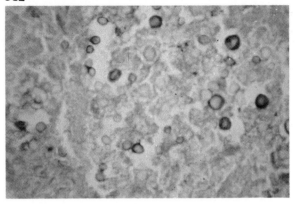

312 Cryptococcus neoformans in lung nodule. Numerous fungal cells are demonstrated. *(PAS stain ×360)*

313 Multiple cryptococcal abscesses in lung. This patient was receiving steroids for lupus erythematosus. Chronic pulmonary cryptococcosis frequently heals without treatment leaving lung fibrosis. Intravenous amphotericin B and oral 5-fluorocytosine are effective treatment.

313

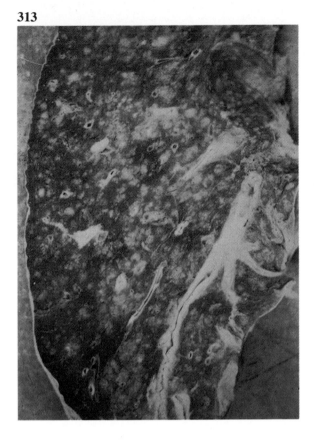

314

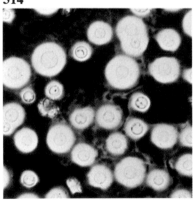

314 Cryptococcus neoformans demonstrated by India ink 'negative' stain of cerebrospinal fluid sediment. The patient had chronic fluctuating cryptococcal meningoencephalitis, which is ultimately fatal in all untreated patients. *(×550)*

315

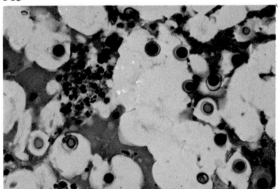

315 Cryptococcus neoformans in brain – necropsy specimen. Oval or round relatively thin-walled cells of varying size are seen in circular clear spaces. The spaces represent the capsule polysaccharide that lacks affinity with the stain.

Aspergillus fumigatus

Aspergillus fumigatus, a ubiquitous mould of decaying vegetation causes a variety of respiratory disorders. The fungi liberate an abundance of respirable-sized spores which inevitably reach the respiratory tract but seldom cause disease. Aspergillosis refers to the diseases caused by the fungus which may present in the following forms:

1 Allergic bronchopulmonary aspergillosis, characterised by asthma, mucous plugs and fleeting eosinophilic pulmonary consolidation often superimposed upon pre-existing extrinsic asthma.
2 Aspergilloma with fungal colonisation of chronic lung cavities.
3 Locally invasive aspergillosis with pulmonary necrosis.
4 Disseminated aspergillosis occurring in the immunosuppressed usually with fatal outcome.

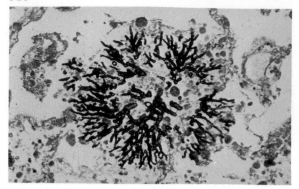

316   Aspergillus species occur as a profusion of dichotomously branching filaments in tissues, exudates or sputum. Note the characteristic radial or 'sunburst' arrangement of the mycelium. *(H&E ×100)*

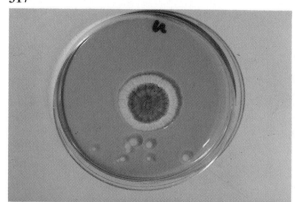

317   Aspergillus fumigatus. Grey-green colonies with a central dome of conidiophores. Sabouraud's medium incubated at 37°C to 40°C.

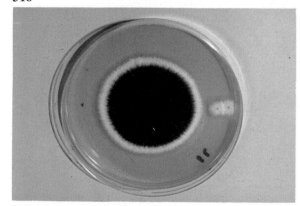

318   Aspergillus niger. Black colonies. Sabouraud's medium incubated at 37°C to 40°C. This species is responsible for chronic ear infections.

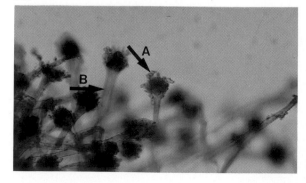

319   Aspergillus fumigatus. Squash preparation stained with methylene blue. The spores develop at the flask-shaped ends of conidiophores and on culture appear as a raised smooth mass that is green in colour. Sporing conidiophores may be seen in tissue from lung cavities (A = spores; B = conidiophores).

Allergic bronchopulmonary aspergillosis

320

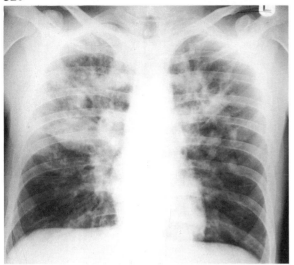

321

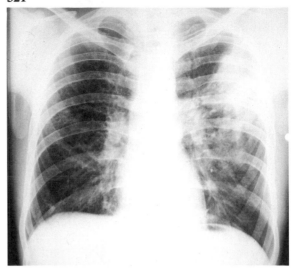

320 Allergic bronchopulmonary aspergillosis. Widespread non-segmental predominantly upper-zone shadows caused by eosinophilic pneumonia in a long-standing case of allergic aspergillosis. Malaise and fever are usual although this patient was symptom free. A peripheral blood eosinophilia accompanies the pulmonary consolidation.

321 Allergic bronchopulmonary aspergillosis. Spontaneous clearing of most of the shadowing seen in **320** within one month. The fleeting nature of the shadowing is often emphasised but fixed abnormal shadows may be found. Mucous impaction by bronchial plugs harbouring mycelial elements of the fungus blocks a segment of the left upper lobe.

322

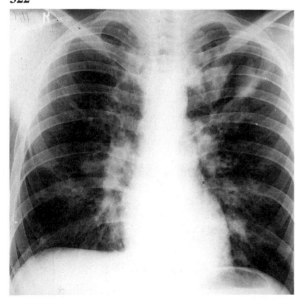

323

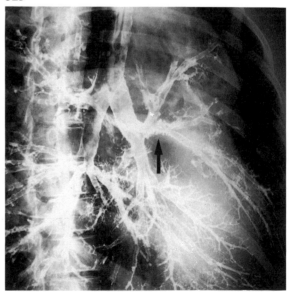

322 Allergic bronchopulmonary aspergillosis. Clearing of shadowing seen in **321** with corticosteroids. The mucous plug seen in the left upper zone was expectorated. Recurrent attacks leave in their wake a characteristic pattern of proximal bronchiectasis.

323 Bronchogram from a patient with bronchopulmonary aspergillosis showing proximal bronchiectasis. Bronchial wall damage may occur where mucous plugs have occluded the bronchi to produce tissue damage (arrowed). Type III reactivity is evident from bronchial-wall damage, pulmonary infiltrate, delayed-type skin tests, precipitating antibodies and elevated serum aspergillus-specific IgG. The presence of granulomas in bronchi and lung indicate cell-mediated Type IV reactivity.

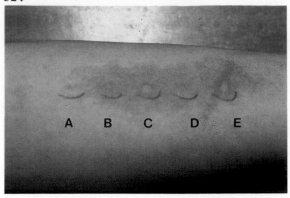

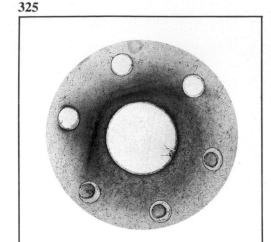

324 Skin prick sensitivity to aspergillus. Asthma is the commonest disorder associated with A. fumigatus, and sensitisation is most frequent in atopic individuals with coincident sensitivity to pollens or dust. Aspergillus fumigatus colonises the bronchial tree giving rise to a complex series of immunological reactions, and presenting with asthma, eosinophilia and pulmonary infiltrates. Aspergillus is found in sputum and bronchial washings. The eosinophilia, asthma, elevated serum IgE levels, aspergillus-specific IgE and positive immediate-type skin test all reflect Type I reactivity. (A: Control; B: House dust mite; C: Grass pollen; D: Tree pollen; E: Aspergillus fumigatus.)

325 Allergic bronchopulmonary aspergillosis – precipitin arcs. Precipitating antibodies may be identified in the serum of two-thirds of patients with allergic aspergillosis. The number of precipitin arcs varies from one to three. Aspergillus antigen extracts are placed in the peripheral agar wells and the patient's serum in the central well. As diffusion occurs through the agar-disc, lines of precipitate form in the region where the serum antibodies and extract antigen are in optimal concentration.

This stained preparation exhibits three 'weak' precipitin lines directed against two of the antigens. (Ouchterlony's method.)

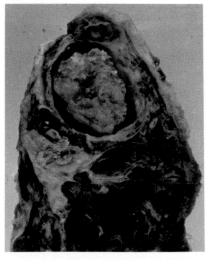

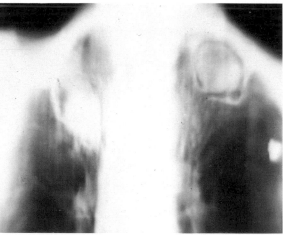

326 Aspergilloma (mycetoma). One of the special features of A. fumigatus is that it is able to maintain growth within the lung. The mycelium grows within pre-existing bullae or cavities or areas of destroyed lung.

327 Bilateral apical pulmonary aspergillomas. Note the transradiant halo of air surrounding the fungus ball (mycetoma) in this tomogram.

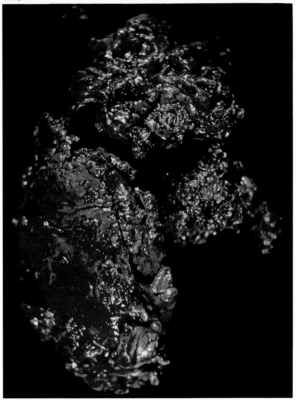

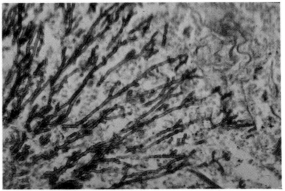

329 Invasive pulmonary aspergillosis in an immuno-suppressed patient receiving cytotoxic treatment for leukaemia.

The branched septate hyphae 4 to 5 μm wide are variably stained and some show characteristic dichotomous branching. *(H&E ×100)*

328 A typical aspergilloma consists of a mass of mycelium lying within a pulmonary cavity.

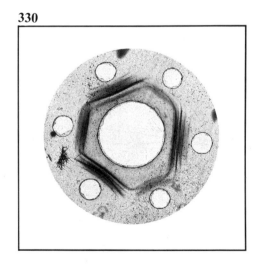

330 Aspergilloma. Precipitins with many arcs are usually demonstrated. Skin tests to Aspergillus fumigatus are unlikely to be positive. The immune reaction fades and the precipitins usually become negative when a mycetoma is removed.

The test serum shows five or six precipitin lines directed against four of the aspergillus antigens. (Ouchterlony's method, Amido Schwartz stain, transmitted light.)

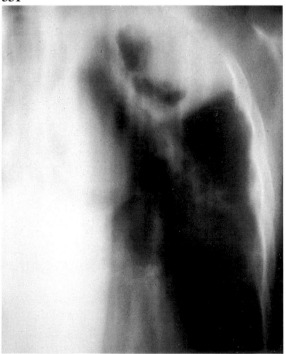

331 A carcinoma in the left upper lobe cavitated to give an appearance simulating a mycetoma. However, there is no transradiant halo. The diagnosis was made by percutaneous needle biopsy.

Histoplasmosis

Histoplasmosis occurs in many parts of the world and is endemic in the central and eastern states of the USA. In endemic areas asymptomatic infection is common but disability rare.

Histoplasma capsulatum, the causative organism, contaminates bird and bat droppings. The disease is usually transmitted by inhaling dust from such sources. The initial respiratory infection is followed by widespread dissemination to the reticuloendothelial system. H. capsulatum is almost exclusively an intracellular parasite.

332

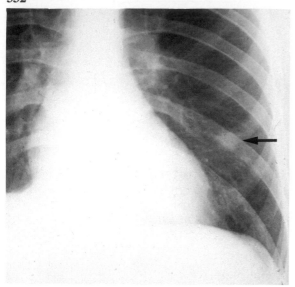

333

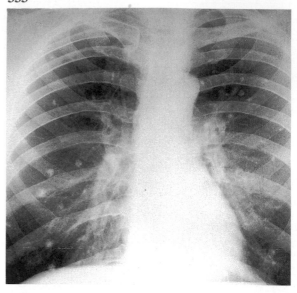

332 Primary pulmonary histoplasmosis. Primary contact with H. capsulatum may result in a transient influenza-like respiratory tract infection, or less commonly pneumonia. This patient had a 'viral pneumonia' after exploring caves in S. America. One month later there was a small primary lesion in the left lower lobe and left hilar lymph node enlargement; a histoplasmin skin test became positive. The primary lesion and associated hilar lymphadenopathy are reminiscent of the primary complex of tuberculosis.

333 Primary pulmonary histoplasmosis. Healing with residual fibrosis and multiple calcified lesions may follow a protracted course.

334

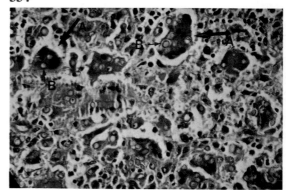

334 A chronic granuloma caused by H. capsulatum. The reticuloendothelial system is particularly involved by histoplasma infection, with fever, lymphadenopathy, splenomegaly and anaemia. Granulomas may develop in the tissues (arrowed A). H. capsulatum lies within numerous foreign body giant cells (arrowed B).

335

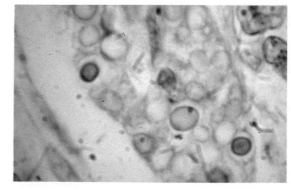

335 Histoplasma capsulatum in lung. Spherical, uninuclear yeast cells with irregularly distributed cytoplasm and thick double-contoured walls. The cell wall stains poorly, giving the impression of a capsule. (*H&E ×1000*)

Hydatid disease

Hydatid disease is due to infection with the ova of Echinococcus granulosus. Ova excreted from the dog, the primary host, develop into hydatid cysts in the liver and lungs of secondary hosts – sheep, cattle, pigs or camels. Ingested ova burrow through the wall of the intestine, to enter the portal circulation and then pass on to the liver. About 10 to 20 per cent of ova may pass through the liver and impact in vessels in the lung. Hydatid cysts are frequently multiple. The life cycle of the echinococcus is completed when the dog ingests diseased organs from the secondary hosts. Man is usually infected by handling dogs.

Pulmonary hydatid cysts may be detected by chance or with features of a lung abscess. Rarely hydatids may rupture with acute expectoration of salty hydatid cyst fluid-containing scolices.

The radiographic appearance varies, for some cysts appear as a solid mass while in others a crescent of air is visible between the hydatid and compressed surrounding lung – the 'pulmonary meniscus' sign. When hydatid pulmonary disease is suspected a Casoni test or complement fixation test should be performed to avoid diagnostic needling.

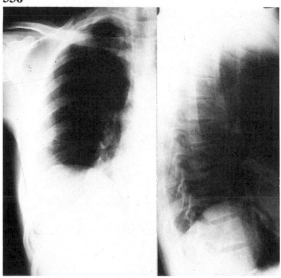

336   Hydatid cysts. A circular opacity is visible in the right lower lobe of a 30 year old sheep farmer. Endemic areas include the Middle East, India, South America, Wales, Australia and New Zealand.

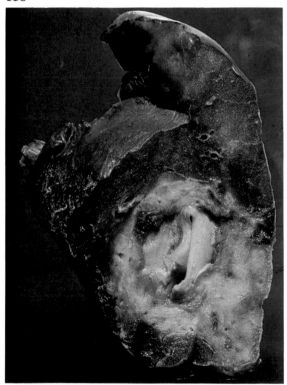

338   Lobectomy specimen showing a large hydatid cyst. Note the thin, white adventitial layer of cyst and the surrounding pneumonia.

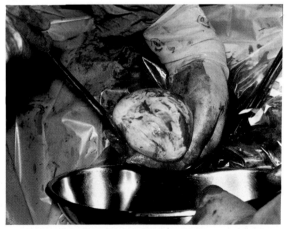

337   Surgical enucleation of a large hydatid cyst from right lung. Simple cysts may be removed along with the adventitial membrane. At operation it is important to protect the pleura from contamination by spilt cyst fluid. Larger or complicated cysts may require segmental or lobar resection.

339

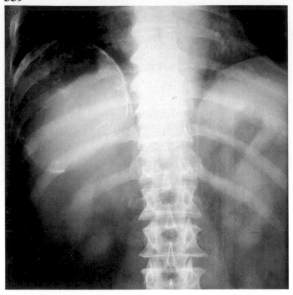

339 Calcified hepatic hydatid cyst. When the chest physician suspects pulmonary hydatid disease, a liver scan is worthwhile because these cysts are multisystem.

340

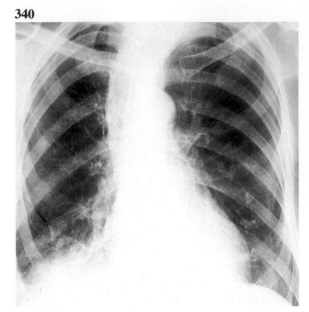

340 Cholangiopulmonary fistula caused by rupture of a hepatic hydatid cyst into a right lower lobe bronchus.

341

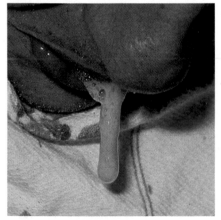

341 Cholangiopulmonary fistula.
Yellow frothy bile-stained sputum.

342

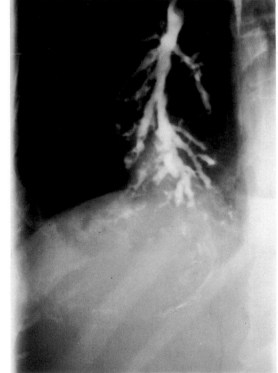

342 Cholangiopulmonary fistula. Radio-opaque dye outlining a large hepatic hydatid-cyst cavity which drains into bronchi in the right lower lobe (same patient as **340**).

Opportunistic infections

It is no longer sufficient to recognise the causal organism of a respiratory infection and treat it with an appropriate antibiotic. Today it is also important to assess the background factors which allow the infection to establish itself in a poor soil. The patient's resistance to infection may be impoverished by poor cellular (T cell) or humoral (B cell) immunity, poor defensive macrophages, transplantation, immunosuppressive drug regimens, heroin, alcoholism and malnutrition. This allows a variety of exotic organisms to cause not only respiratory infections but also widespread septicaemia.

Table: Opportunistic infections in the immunosuppressed.

Mechanism	Defect	Type of infection
Poor cell-mediated immunity Ineffective T-cell defence	Renal transplant recipients	Cytomegalovirus, Pneumocystis, Listeria monocytogenes, Candida albicans
	Bone marrow transplant recipients	Cytomegalovirus
	Elderly Alcoholic Diabetic	Tuberculosis
	Hodgkin's disease	Cryptococcus; Pneumocystis; Coccidioides Varicella-zoster
	Neoplasia treated with chemotherapy	Cytomegalovirus Pneumocystis
	Newborn	Candida albicans Pneumocystis
	Extensive burns	Staphylococcus aureus Pseudomonas aeruginosa
	Heroin addiction	Staphylococcal lung abscess HBsAg
	Prolonged corticosteroid therapy	Pneumocystis Aspergillus

(continued)

Mechanism	Defect	Type of infection
Poor humoral immunity Ineffective B-cells	Hypogammaglobulinaemia	Herpes zoster; Mycoplasma; Giardia; Campylobacter
	Myelomatosis	Pneumococcus
Poor humoral immunity	Leukaemia	Aspergillus; Pseudomonas Pneumocystis; Phycomycetes
	Sickle-cell disease	Mycoplasma; S. paratyphi
	Splenectomy	Pneumococcus
Poor phagocytosis	Chronic granulomatous disease of childhood	S. aureus Gram-negative enteric bacilli
	Neutropenia	Gram-negative bacilli Pseudomonas
	Aplastic anaemia	Pseudomonas S. aureus
Poor local macrophage function	Cystic fibrosis	Pseudomonas S. aureus
	Alveolar proteinosis	Nocardia asteroides
	Pneumoconiosis	Atypical mycobacteria
	Assisted ventilation and nebulisers	Pseudomonas Serratia Flavobacterium
Foreign body	Indwelling catheter	Escherichia coli Penicillinase-producing S. aureus
	Heart valve replacement	S. viridans S. aureus Gram-negative bacilli

Pneumocystis

343

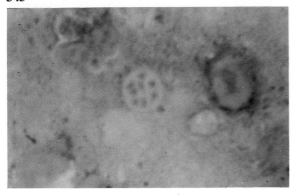

344

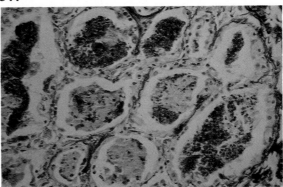

343 Pneumocystis carinii. Cysts approximately $5\,\mu m$ in diameter containing up to eight oval bodies called sporozoites are diagnostic. Pneumocystis carinii is distributed worldwide. It resembles a protozoa-like cyst in appearance, although it is related to fungi. Exact classification is difficult for antifungal agents are not beneficial to patients with pneumocystis infection while the disease reverses with antiprotozoal chemotherapy. It is an infection of the immunosuppressed patient.

344 Pneumocystis carinii. The alveoli are filled with amorphous exudate containing plasma cells and organisms. Necrosis and tissue invasion are conspicuously absent. The organisms are seldom seen on sputum examination and diagnosis is usually made from the presence of pneumocystis in a biopsy specimen or from exudate obtained by bronchial lavage.

345

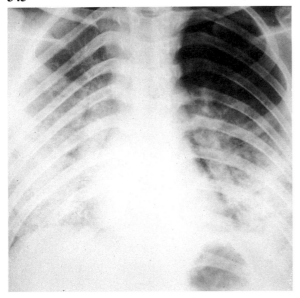

346

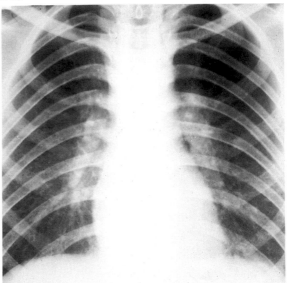

345 and 346 Pneumocystis carinii. The xray shows a bilateral 'groundglass' appearance in the mid zone; it resolved with sulphonamide-trimethoprim therapy.

Cytomegalovirus (CMV)

Cytomegalovirus is a DNA virus indistinguishable from herpes simplex. Congenital infection may result in the death of the foetus in utero and it is estimated that one in every 1000 infants is retarded by CNS damage. Silent infection in children and young adults is common and CMV antibody titres are frequently elevated. Two per cent of young adults, ten per cent of pregnant women and 50 per cent of immunosuppressed renal-transplant patients excrete cytomegalovirus. Cytomegalovirus pneumonia or hepatitis occurs in immunosuppressed patients. Latent infection may be reactivated or may be acquired from transplants or blood transfusions.

347

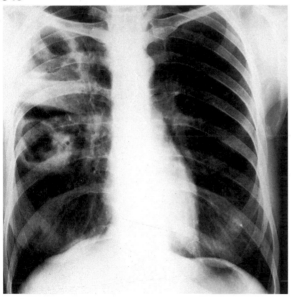

347 Cytomegalovirus. Prominent intranuclear and intracytoplasmic inclusions are seen. A diffuse pneumonia similar to that found in pneumocystis infections may occur. Hepatosplenomegaly is common in CMV infection but does not occur with pneumocystis infection.

Staphylococcal lung abscesses

348

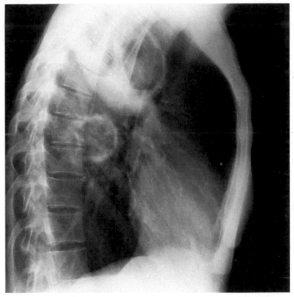

348 Staphylococcal lung abscess. Two large cavities are present in the right lung. This heroin addict presented with a cough, chest pain and fever. The sputum was purulent.

349

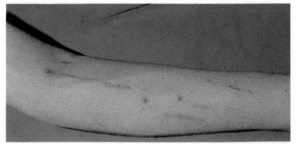

349 Staphylococcal lung abscess. Lateral view of **348**.

350

350 Staphylococcal lung abscess. Multiple injection sites were present all over accessible veins. Intravenous injections of contaminated fluid are common in addicts. This man injected water obtained from lavatory pans.

Impaired cell-mediated immunity

351

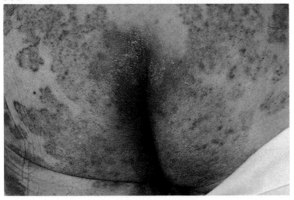

351 Chronic cutaneous candida infection.

352

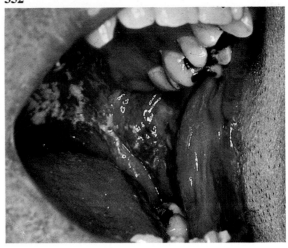

352 Oral candidiasis.

Impaired humoral immunity

353

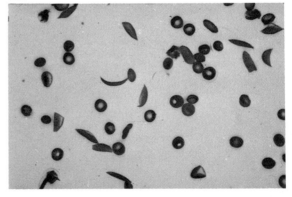

353 Sickle-cell disease may be associated with an increased predisposition to infection. Bone infarction may lead to Salmonella osteomyelitis and splenic infarction to S. pneumoniae septicaemia.

354

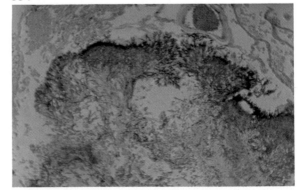

354 Invasive aspergillosis in the lungs of a patient receiving cytotoxic chemotherapy for leukaemia. Fatal dissemination to the meninges and other organs may occur.

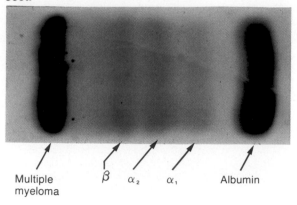

355a

Multiple myeloma β α₂ α₁ Albumin

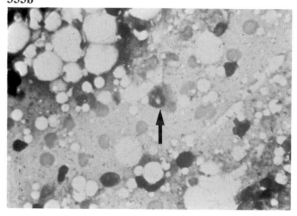

355b

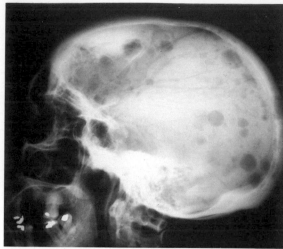

356

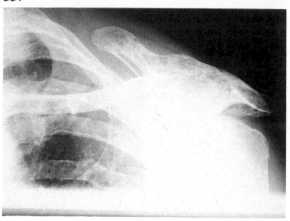

357

355a and b Multiple myeloma. Cellulose acetate electrophoresis showing a band of abnormal globulin. The bone marrow is infiltrated by abnormal plasma cells.

356 and 357 Multiple myelomatosis with 'punched out' lytic bone cysts in the skull and clavicles. The clue to diagnosis was recurrent chest infections caused by humoral depression.

358 Fatal vaccinia with pneumonia in a patient given smallpox vaccination before visiting Europe. She was immunosuppressed by cytotoxic drugs for chronic lymphatic leukaemia.

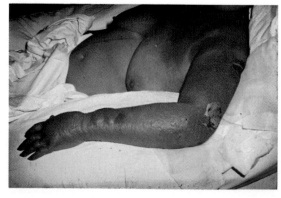

358

17 Immunological lung injury

Certain respiratory disorders and their systemic counterparts can be explained by Gell-Coombs' types I, II, III or IV reactivity (see Table). But it is increasingly recognised that some respiratory diseases are caused by a complex interplay of more than one of these mechanisms. In these types of lung injury there is increasing recognition of the part played by T and B cells.

Table: Gell-Coombs' types of mechanisms of lung injury.

Immune type	I	II	III	IV
Alternative name	Immediate hypersensitivity	Cytotoxic antibody	Antigen-antibody immune complex	Delayed-type cell-mediated
Cell types involved	B Mast cell Basophil Eosinophil	B or K Macrophage	B Polymorphs Platelets	T Macrophage Giant and epithelioid
Immunoglobulin	IgE	IgG; IgM	IgG	
Clinical disorder – respiratory	Asthma Hay fever Rhinitis	Goodpasture's syndrome	Sarcoidosis Erythema nodosum Rheumatoid lung Rheumato-pneumoconiosis Fibrosing alveolitis	Sarcoidosis Nitrofurantoin lung Allergic alveolitis Bronchopulmonary aspergillosis Wegener's granulomatosis Churg-Strauss syndrome
– systemic	Conjunctivitis Urticaria	Glomerulo-nephritis	Serum sickness Systemic lupus erythematosus Uveitis; scleritis Retinal vasculitis Behçet's syndrome	Graft rejection Contact dermatitis Phacoantigenic uveitis Phlyctenular conjunctivitis Interstitial keratitis
Diagnostic measurements	Immediate skin tests Raised blood and mucosal IgE	Immuno-fluorescence reveals linear IgG in alveolar and renal basement membrane	Circulating immune complexes Complement conversion High ESR Immunofluorescence	Skin tests Lymphocyte transformation Macrophage-migration inhibition Cell-mediated cytotoxicity Colony inhibition
Treatment – steroids	Yes	Yes	Yes	Yes
– other	Sodium cromoglycate	Plasmapheresis	Immunosuppressives and immunostimulants	Immunosuppressives

Table: Respiratory disorders in which there is a complex interplay of immune mechanisms.

Respiratory disorder	Type of immune mechanism involved			
	I	II	III	IV
Bronchopulmonary aspergillosis	+		+	?+
Extrinsic allergic alveolitis	?+		+	+
Wegener's granulomatosis			+	+
Churg-Strauss syndrome	+		?+	+
Sarcoidosis			+	+

Table: Properties of serum immunoglobulins.

Immuno-globulin	Serum concentration (mg/ml)	Intravascular (percentage)	Molecular weight	Produced by foetus	Special properties
IgG	12	45	150000 (7S)		General purpose antibody against infections (secondary response) Placenta transfer Complement-fixing
IgA	2	42	160000 (7–13)		Principal Ig in external secretions Some natural isohaemagglutinins
IgM	1.2	80	890000 (19S)	Yes	Natural isohaemagglutinins Primary antibody response Complement-fixing
IgD	0.03	75	178000 (7–8S)		Biological activity not known ? Lymphocyte antigen receptor
IgE	0.00004	51	187000 (7–9S)	Yes	Reaginic antibody Present in external secretions

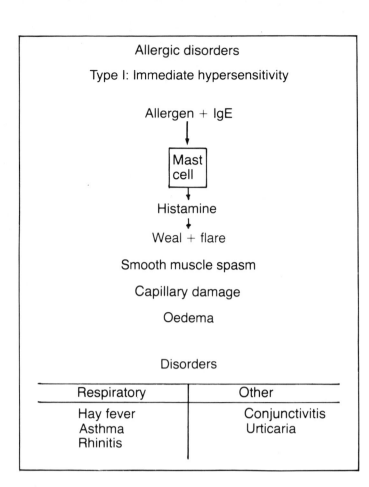

Allergic disorders

Type I: Immediate hypersensitivity

Allergen + IgE

Mast cell

Histamine

Weal + flare

Smooth muscle spasm

Capillary damage

Oedema

Disorders

Respiratory	Other
Hay fever	Conjunctivitis
Asthma	Urticaria
Rhinitis	

Bronchial asthma

Although there is no universally accepted definition, bronchial asthma may be defined as 'a disorder of function characterised by dyspnoea caused by widespread narrowing of peripheral airways in the lungs, varying in severity over short periods of time either spontaneously or with treatment'.

Asthma is a common condition. The prevalence of recurrent wheezing in UK pre-school children is estimated at seven to eight per cent and in schoolchildren from two to five per cent.

Airway narrowing may be caused by a variety of precipitating factors including hypersensitivity to inhaled allergens, respiratory infections, exercise, drugs, emotional factors and non-specific irritants such as smoke, gases or changes in temperature of inspired air.

Clinically it is convenient to divide asthmatics into two major subgroups:

1 *Extrinsic asthma*. This usually begins early in life, especially affecting males. Patients show positive immediate hypersensitivity to skin prick tests and also show a high incidence of seasonal rhinitis, and flexural eczema.

2 *Intrinsic asthma*. Typical in middle-aged adults, especially females. Recognisable allergic features are absent.

Patients in either group may be susceptible to the same aggravating factors and may respond to the same treatment.

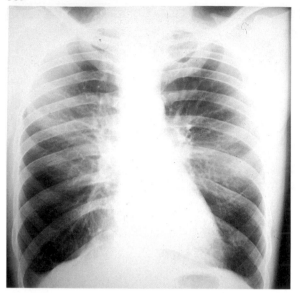

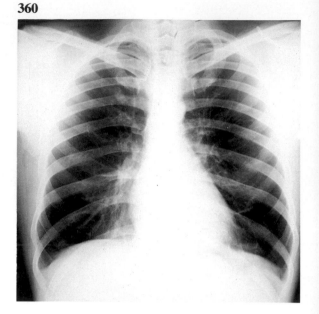

359   Acute attack of asthma. The radiological signs at presentation are those of hyperinflation. The rib cage silhouette is 'square' and the sides of the thorax parallel. The diaphragms are depressed to the level of the 11th rib, the muscle reflections of the right diaphragm are visible and the upper lobe blood vessels are distended.

360   Asthma. The same patient as in **359** on the 8th day of treatment. The ribcage silhouette is normal. Peak expiratory flow chart shows improvement with treatment.

361

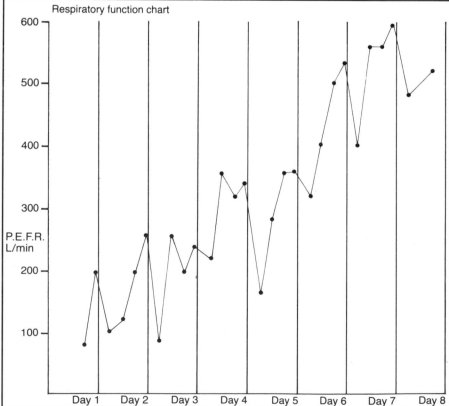

361   Peak expiratory flow chart in asthma (same patient as in **359**). Treatment with parenteral corticosteroids and ß₂ stimulants on admission. This patient suffered from pollen allergy and became acutely wheezy while on holiday in a farming area.

Respiratory function chart

P.E.F.R. L/min

Day 1   Day 2   Day 3   Day 4   Day 5   Day 6   Day 7   Day 8

362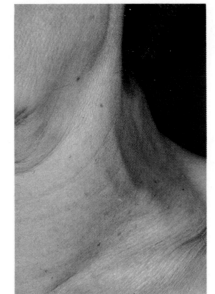

363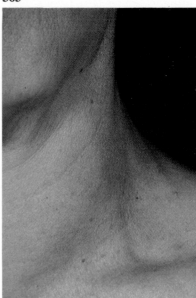

362 and 363 Asthma – the jugular venous pulsation. The large intrathoracic pressure swings seen in severe asthma cause corresponding variations in the venous pressure.

The jugular venous pressure is high during expiration (**362**) with filling of the neck veins. On inspiration the neck veins empty (**363**).

364

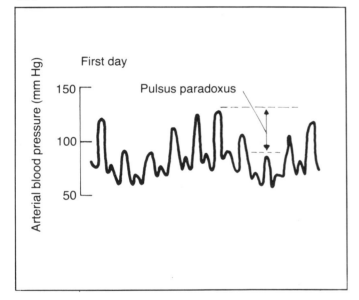

365

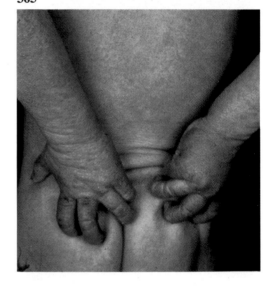

364 Pulsus paradoxus. The arterial pressure trace shows a variation in pressure of 30 mm Hg between inspiration and expiration.

Pulsus paradoxus is defined as more than a 10 per cent or 10 mm Hg fall in systolic pressure with inspiration. It is an exaggeration of the normal finding of decreased arterial pressure with inspiration.

This sign reflects large expiratory pressures found in both severe asthma and severe fixed air-flow obstruction.

365 Childhood eczema. Itchy eczematous lesions which become excoriated and secondarily infected. A family history of atopy, extrinsic asthma or rhinitis is common.

366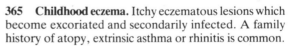

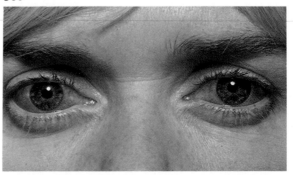

366 Conjunctivitis caused by grass-pollen allergy in a young atopic hay-fever sufferer. Immunotherapy with a series of desensitisation injections of aqueous grass-pollen extract improved this patient's severe seasonal symptoms.

367

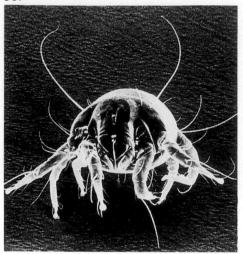

368

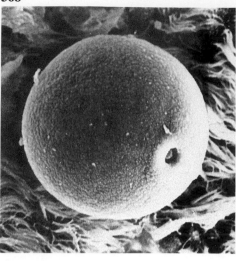

367 Dermatophagoides: the house dust mite. Two main species are responsible for allergic symptoms. D. pteronyssinus in Europe and D. Farinae in the Middle East and North America. The mite survives upon sequestrated human skin scales in moist temperate environments. Mattresses and bed linen are often infested and provide the link between mite allergy and nocturnal symptoms in the sensitive individual. The allergic symptoms are most severe from November to January at the time of most intense mite activity.

368 Grass pollen grain against background of ciliated epithelium of rat. The severity of rhinitis, hay fever and grass-pollen asthma is related to the quantitative seasonal counts of pollen grains in the atmosphere. The most common varieties of grass pollen are the crested dog's tail, fescue, foxtail, meadow rye, timothy, cocksfoot and brome.

The nature of the pollen varies with geographical regions: pollen from the rag weed in the USA, the prosopis species of tree in the Middle East and the mulberry along the Mediterranean coast are especially common causes of allergy. *(EM ×1500)*

369

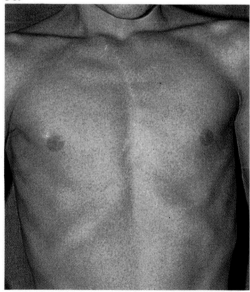

369 Chronic asthma in childhood results in delayed growth. The chest is hyperinflated and the lower ribs and costal margin splayed out – the deformity is called Harrison's sulcus. Children with chronic asthma tend to be stunted. This ten-year-old child with perennial asthma suffered retardation of growth.

370 Pollen chart (page 135). The pollen count is obtained by sampling air sucked through a special chamber which deposits the pollen grains onto a sticky glass plate. The plate is examined after 24 hours and the count of pollen grains is expressed as the number of grains per cubic metre of air. A count of 50 pollen grains per cubic metre of air can cause discomfort to sensitised individuals.

Different plants produce pollen at different times of the year. Symptoms are most commonly caused by the airborne pollens liberated from trees, grass and nettles.

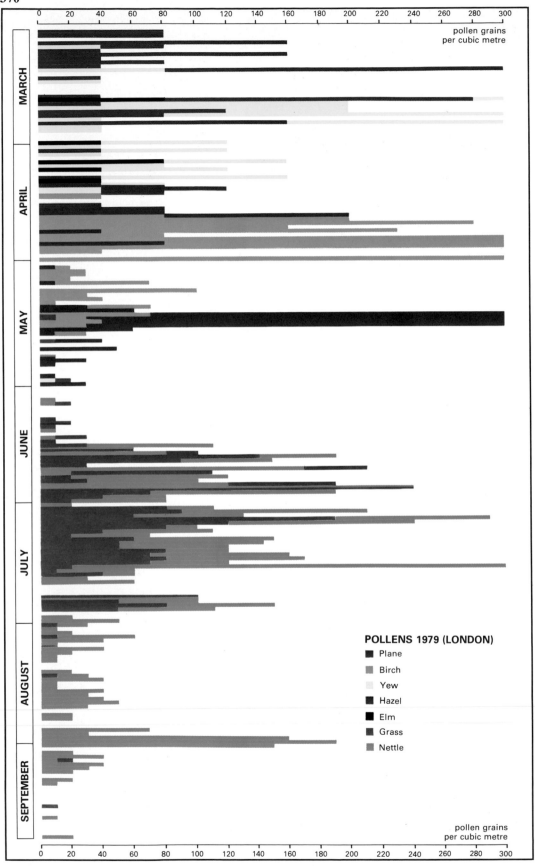

POLLENS 1979 (LONDON)

- ■ Plane
- ■ Birch
- ■ Yew
- ■ Hazel
- ■ Elm
- ■ Grass
- ■ Nettle

pollen grains
per cubic metre

371a
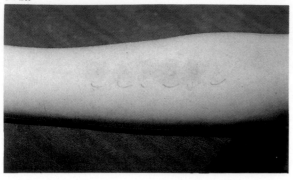

371b
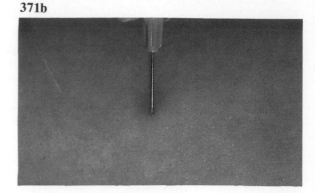

371a Immediate skin-prick test reactions showing wheals, pseudopodia and surrounding flares. The antigen reacts with a specific class of antibody bound to mast cells or circulating basophils which leads to the release of vasoactive amines. The reaction is maximal at 15 to 20 minutes, and fades in 60 to 90 minutes. Provided the control test is negative, any wheal surrounded by erythema, regardless of size, constitutes a positive test. The size of the wheal does not correlate with the severity of symptoms.

Two classes of mast-cell sensitising antibody are recognised; reaginic IgE antibody (long-term homocytotropic antibody) and IgG antibody (short-term sensitising antibody).

371b The technique of skin-prick testing. The point of a small-gauge needle is passed through a drop of allergen into the superficial layers of the skin. This introduces about 10^{-6} ml of antigen. Blood should not be drawn. Immediate reactions to prick tests correlate closely with measurements of specific IgE.

372
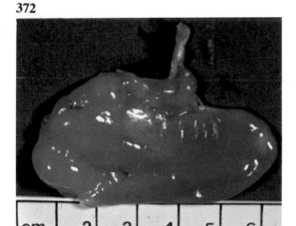

372—Nasal polyp. Polyps are more common in asthmatics than normal controls. Nasal polypi and aspirin sensitivity are most common in intrinsic asthmatic patients.

373
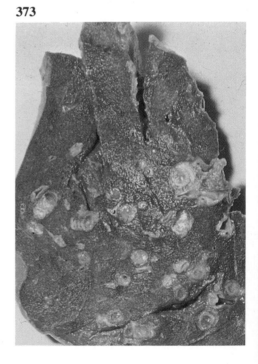

373 Plugs of very viscid mucus project from the lumen of the sectioned bronchi. Lung from a fatal case of asthma.

374

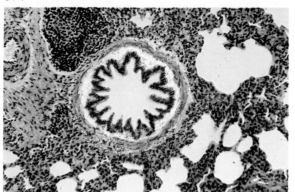

374 Section of bronchiole in asthma with narrowing of the lumen caused by constriction of smooth muscle. Lung tissue from asthmatics shows hypertrophy of smooth muscle in the bronchial walls, thickening of the mucosa with hypertrophy of the mucus glands and eosinophilic infiltration. Mucus plugs may block the airways.

375

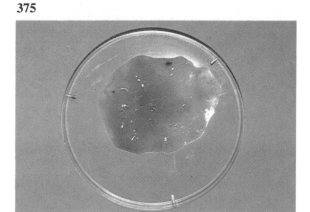

375 Sputum specimen in asthma. Thick gelatinous sputum containing eosinophils and other cell debris in inspissated mucus.

376

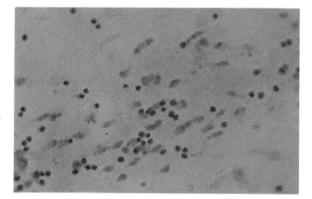

376 Sputum eosinophilia in asthma is a common diagnostic feature. Large numbers of eosinophils may be present in sputum and nasal secretions. Stain for eosinophils by air-drying a thin smear; fix with methyl alcohol for three minutes; flood slide with Jenner's stain diluted with distilled water for five minutes, rinse and air dry. Count eosinophils and express as percentage of total leucocytes. They may be present in abundance in asthma, hay fever, aspergillus infection and parasitic infestation.

377

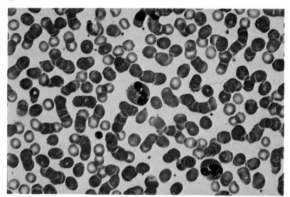

377 Blood eosinophilia is a non-specific feature of asthma which usually occurs in association with sputum eosinophilia.

Table: Occupational asthma.

Industrial exposure	Provoking material	Skin test	Diagnostic tests Bronchial provocation	Specific serum IgE
Animal contact Farmers Veterinarians Poultry breeders Fishermen Laboratory workers	Bird, fish, animal, insect – dander – secretions – serum – pigeon bloom	+	+	+
Bakers	Flour	+	+	+
Grain elevator operators	Grain	+	+	+
Pharmaceutical	Ampicillin	+	+	
	Formalin		+	
	Phenylglycine acid chloride	+	+	
	Sulphone chloramide	+	+	
Textile	Cotton dust	+	+	
Carpenters	Wood dust	+	+	
Printers	Vegetable gums	+		
Metal	Platinum	+	+	+
	Nickel	+	+	
Plastic and resin electronics	Ethylene diamine	+	+	
	Phthalic anhydride	+	+	+
	Trimellitic anhydride	+	+	+
	Hog trypsin	+	+	
	Colophony resin flux		+	
Detergent	Enzymes from Bacillus subtilis	+	+	+
Food	Castor bean	+	+	+
	Green coffee bean	+	+	+
	Papain	+	+	+
	Pancreatic extracts	+	+	
Chemical	Ammonia, sulphur dioxide, hydrochloric acid, chlorine, nitrogen dioxide, toluene, di-isocyanate		+	

Adapted from R. J. Davies, 'Brit. J. Hosp. Med.', Aug. 1979, **22**, **136**.

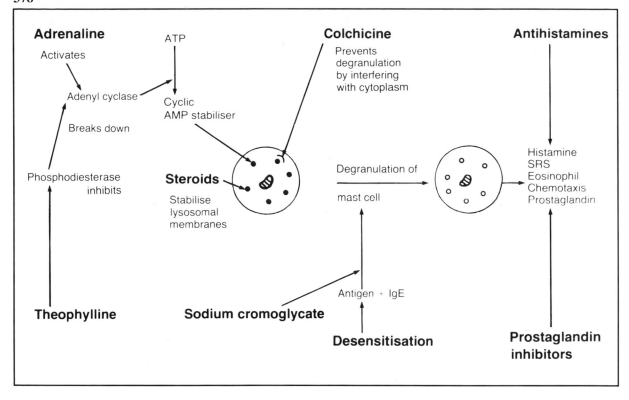

Adrenaline

Activates

ATP

Adenyl cyclase

Cyclic
AMP stabiliser

Breaks down

Phosphodiesterase
inhibits

Theophylline

Colchicine

Prevents
degranulation
by interfering
with cytoplasm

Steroids

Stabilise
lysosomal
membranes

Degranulation of

mast cell

Sodium cromoglycate

Antigen + IgE

Desensitisation

Antihistamines

Histamine
SRS
Eosinophil
Chemotaxis
Prostaglandin

**Prostaglandin
inhibitors**

Eosinophilic pneumonia
(synonyms: simple pulmonary
eosinophilia, Löeffler's syndrome)

Pulmonary disease associated with either blood
or tissue eosinophilia embraces a wide group of
conditions. In some the cause is well established,
such as drug reactions, parasite infestations,
asthma and allergic bronchopulmonary aspergillosis. A tentative association may be assumed
with microfilaria infection in some cases of tropical pulmonary eosinophilia, but in the remainder
the cause is obscure.

The immunological mechanism may not be a
type I reaction but as these conditions often
present with asthmatic symptoms, they are best
considered with asthma.

Eosinophilic pneumonia is characterised by
transient non-segmental radiographic shadows
accompanied by a moderate blood eosinophilia.
Symptoms are mild and may even be absent.

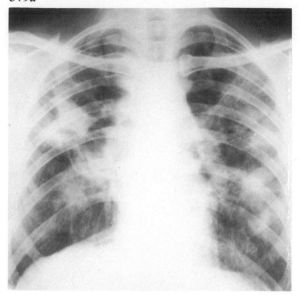

379a

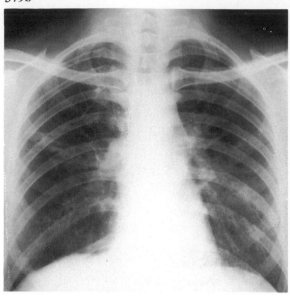

379b

379a Eosinophilic pneumonia (Löeffler's syndrome). Non-segmental transitory shadows tending to be distributed peripherally. The 'reverse pulmonary oedema' pattern is characteristic. The total white cell count was 10,500 per cu mm with 1600 (15 per cent) eosinophils.

379b Löeffler's syndrome. Spontaneous clearing usually occurs within a month. In this case corticosteroids were given with prompt remission of the shadowing seen in **379a**. Symptoms are usually mild and may even be absent.

Chronic eosinophilic pneumonia (synonyms: cryptogenic pulmonary eosinophilia)

380

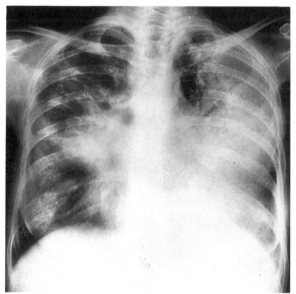

381

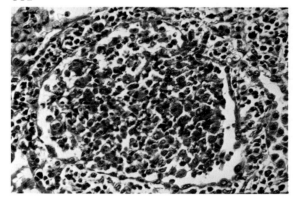

381 Chronic eosinophilic pneumonia. The lung biopsy shows infiltration of the alveolar walls by eosinophils and histiocytes. The alveolar space is filled by an exudate containing eosinophils.

380 Chronic eosinophilic pneumonia. This extensive shadowing cleared with corticosteroid drugs. The typical pattern of 'reversed pulmonary oedema' is more usual. Chronic eosinophilic pneumonia is associated with a constitutional illness in which fever, malaise and weight loss may be accompanied by dyspnoea. Blood eosinophilia may be high but the IgE is only moderately elevated.

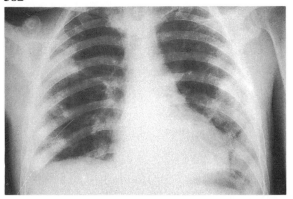

382 Drug-induced pulmonary eosinophilia. This eosinophilic pulmonary infiltrate developed during para-amino salicylic acid therapy for tuberculosis. The infiltrate is typically peripheral and fleeting, resolving to be replaced by other shadows on the same or opposite side. Penicillin, the sulphonamides, tricyclic antidepressants, aspirin, isoniazid, para-amino salicylic acid and even cromolyn sodium are reported to cause transient pulmonary eosinophilia.

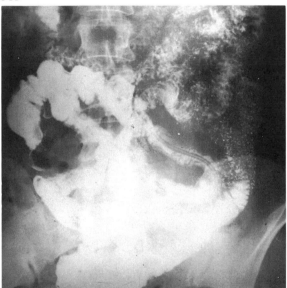

383 Ascariasis (roundworm infestation) and pulmonary eosinophilia. Ascaris lumbricoides is seen in a barium contrast study of the small bowel. Ascaris contains a number of allergenic substances which may induce transient alveolitis and a very elevated blood eosinophil count accompanied by a massive rise in total IgE.

Tropical pulmonary eosinophilia (synonym: pulmonary filariasis)

Tropical pulmonary eosinophilia is closely associated with microfilaria infestation. The clinical features are of asthma with eosinophilia and diffuse bilateral reticulonodular shadowing in the lungs.

385 Blood film of microfilaria (Wuchereria bancrofti). Microfilariae are seldom demonstrated in the blood of patients with tropical eosinophilia and diagnosis is established by the presence of complement-fixing antibodies for filariae and good response to antifilarial medications.

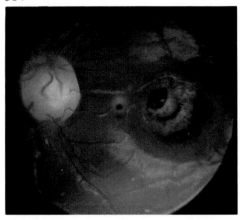

384 Ascaris lumbricoides larva lying in the fundus. Ingested ova release larvae which migrate through the wall of the intestine, pass to the pulmonary circulation and enter the airways before being swallowed to reach maturity in the intestine.

As larvae migrate through the lungs itching, wheezing, dyspnoea and angioneurotic oedema may occur. Some migrating larvae may escape from the lungs into the systemic circulation to be scattered throughout the body. The filariform larvae of other worms may cause similar symptoms.

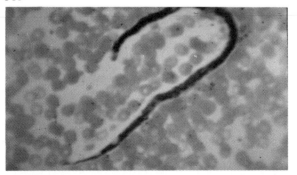

Type II: Cytotoxic antibody-mediated injury

Cell-attached antigen + IgG or IgM antibody

+ Complement

↓

Cell destruction

Cytotoxic antibody cross-reacts with
glomerular and alveolar basement membranes
causing
glomerulonephritis and pulmonary haemorrhage
(Goodpasture's syndrome)

386

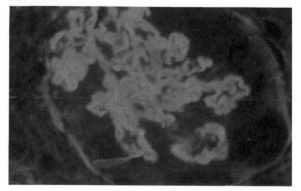

387

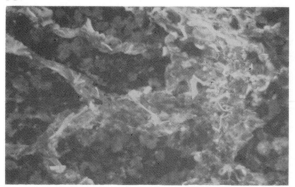

386 and 387 Goodpasture's syndrome. Immuno-fluorescence reveals a linear distribution of IgG globulin along renal and alveolar basement membrane. Recurrent pulmonary haemorrhage, haemoptyses and anaemia are associated with diffuse proliferative glomerulonephritis. Haemosiderin-laden macrophages are found in smears of sputum. Serum antibodies are directed against glomerular basement membrane of the kidney and against alveolar basement membrane of the lung causing injury to the pulmonary capillary bed resulting in pulmonary haemorrhage. The absence of vasculitis and necrotic respiratory tract lesions distinguishes it from Wegener's granulomatosis.

Treatment includes corticosteroids, immunosuppressives and plasmapheresis to remove the circulating antibody.

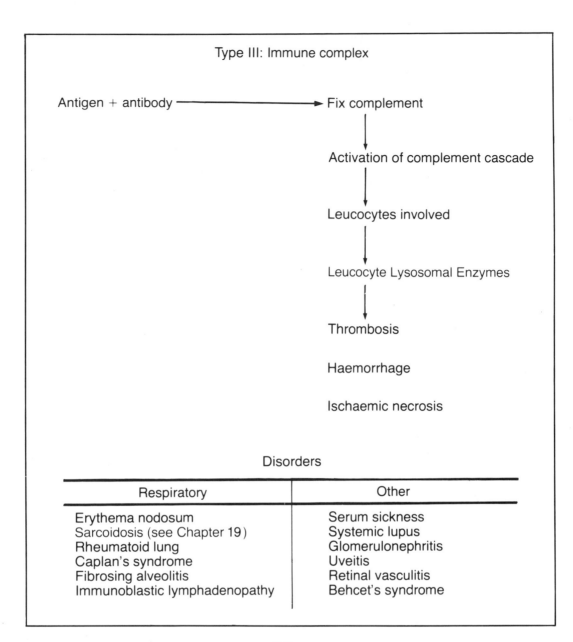

Type III: Immune complex

Antigen + antibody ⟶ Fix complement

Activation of complement cascade

Leucocytes involved

Leucocyte Lysosomal Enzymes

Thrombosis

Haemorrhage

Ischaemic necrosis

Disorders

Respiratory	Other
Erythema nodosum	Serum sickness
Sarcoidosis (see Chapter 19)	Systemic lupus
Rheumatoid lung	Glomerulonephritis
Caplan's syndrome	Uveitis
Fibrosing alveolitis	Retinal vasculitis
Immunoblastic lymphadenopathy	Behcet's syndrome

Rheumatoid lung

Respiratory infection, bronchitis and bronchiectasis are commonplace; lung nodules, apical fibrosis, fibrosing alveolitis, pleural effusions, and pleural thickening also occur frequently. Cryoglobulinaemia and serum Ciq binding activity are negative in uncomplicated rheumatoid arthritis, but positive in three-quarters of those with extra-articular disease, including lung involvement.

388

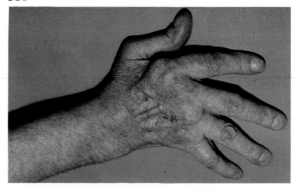

388 Rheumatoid arthritis. The hands at a late stage of the disease.

389

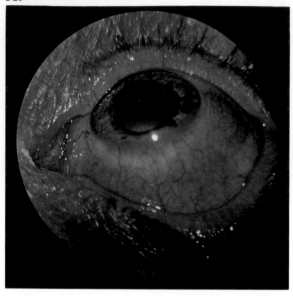

389 Episcleritis indicates activity of the rheumatoid process.

390

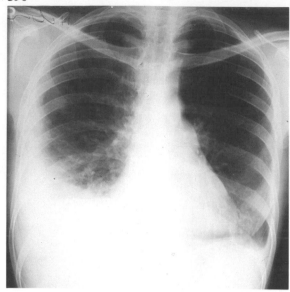

390 Rheumatoid pleural effusion may precede joint symptoms, The fluid contains lymphocytes, a low glucose and high iron content.

391

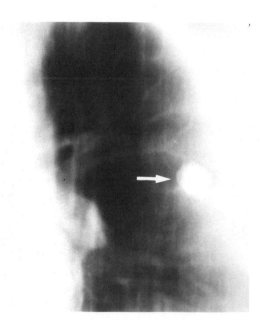

391 Rheumatoid nodules are usually subpleural and more common in men. Biopsy of solitary nodules may be necessary to exclude malignancy. (Tomogram.)

392

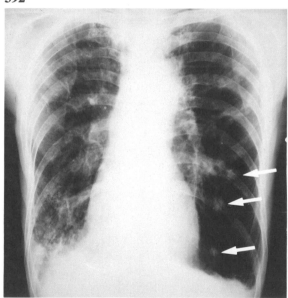

392 Multiple rheumatoid nodules.

393

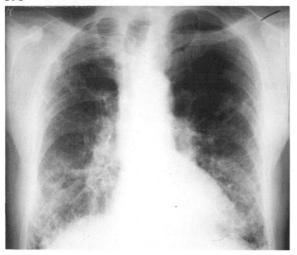

393 Rheumatoid fibrosing alveolitis causes diffuse lower zone shadowing.

394

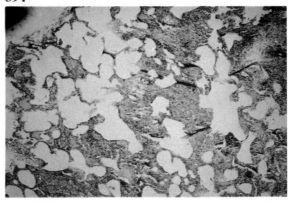

394 Rheumatoid fibrosing alveolitis. Histology reveals thickened alveoli, fibrosis and disorganisation of the lung architecture leading to 'honeycombing'.

Systemic lupus erythematosus (SLE)

This is a chronic multisystem inflammatory disease of unknown cause affecting the skin, joints, kidney, nervous system and serous membranes. It affects females nine times more frequently than males at any age, but most commonly during the 20 to 40 age group. Circulating immune complexes deposit in the lungs and kidneys producing a granular deposition pattern of IgG.

Pleurisy is associated with effusions and with polyarthritis, butterfly skin eruptions, nephritis, neuropsychiatric manifestations, pericarditis or Raynaud's disease. Necrotising renal and cerebral vasculitis carry a poor prognosis.

B cells are overactive producing autoantibodies, whereas T cells are underactive and fail to suppress B cells. The disease occurs particularly in HLA-DRW2 and HLA-DRW3 individuals.

395

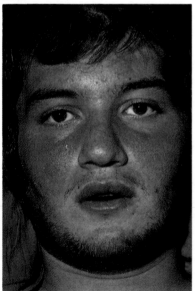

395 The facial butterfly rash is a feature of discoid lupus and is present in about 50 per cent of patients with systemic lupus.

396

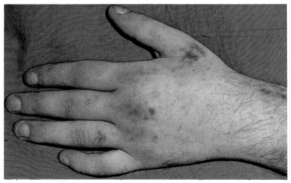

396 Petechial eruption with vasculitis may be caused by tissue deposition of circulating immune complexes.

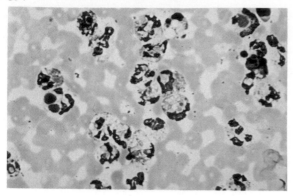

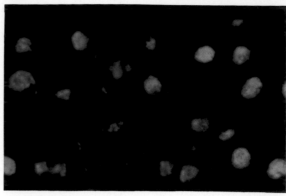

397 Lupus erythematosus cells (LE cells) showing inclusions of nuclear material within the cytoplasm of a polymorphonuclear leucocyte. LE cells are found in 90 per cent of cases of SLE. DNA antibodies are found in 75 per cent and their presence is used as a supporting diagnostic test for SLE.

398 Antinuclear antibody (ANA). These are present in 90 per cent of cases but provide less specific diagnostic information than DNA binding antibodies. The pattern of immunofluorescence is usually diffuse. Other serological characteristics include rheumatoid factor, circulating immune complexes and hypo-complementaemia. (×54 oil)

399

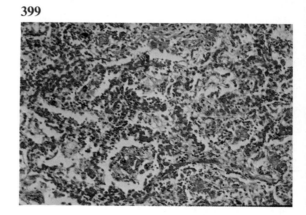

399 Systemic lupus erythematosus. The lung section shows a mixed cellular infiltrate and mild interstitial fibrosis. Pulmonary involvement includes pleurisy with a friction rub or effusion, shifting pulmonary infiltrates, plate atelectasis, and interstitial lung disease; these all lead to hyperventilation, impairment of diffusion capacity and a restrictive pattern of respiration. The lungs, like the kidneys, are vulnerable to immune-complex injury. (H&E ×40)

Pulmonary vasculitis in Behçet's disease

Behçet's disease was originally described as a triad of oral and genital ulceration with relapsing uveitis but is now recognised as a multisystem disease (page 129). The pathology is vasculitis particularly involving the veins. Pulmonary vasculitis may occur as a result of the deposition of circulating antigen-antibody complexes. Cryoglobins of IgM or IgG class are present in 75 per cent of cases. Seronegative arthritis is more evident in patients who are HLA-B27.

400

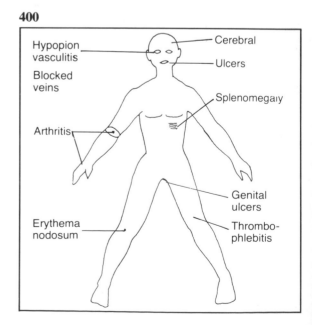

400 Clinical features of Behçet's disease.

401

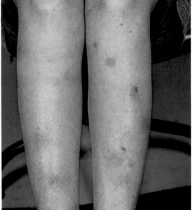

401 Erythema nodosum. Recurrent or chronic erythema nodosum may be found in up to 80 per cent.

402 Chronic genital ulceration. Recurrent ulceration of the scrotum, penile shaft and perineum or haemorrhagic lesions of the glans penis, labia and vaginal mucosa are common.

402

403

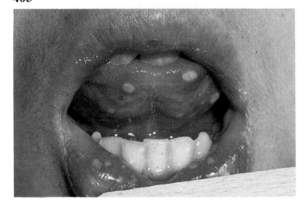

403 Recurrent aphthous stomatitis is most frequent in patients who are HLA-B12. Ulceration of the mouth is virtually a constant feature and similar ulcers may involve the mucosa throughout the alimentary canal.

404

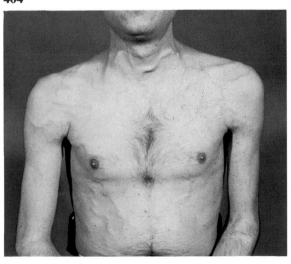

404 Superior and inferior vena caval obstruction in Behçet's disease.

405

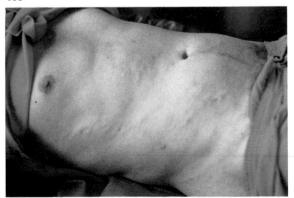

405 Abdominal wall thrombophlebitis. Thrombophlebitis of small and large vessels may be present in up to one-third of patients.

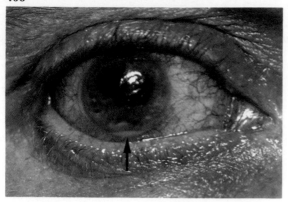

406 Uveitis. Hypopion with fluid level, keratic precipitates and posterior synechiae. Ocular involvement is more frequent in patients who are HLA-B5.

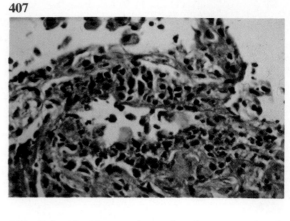

407 Behçet's disease. A small pulmonary vein disrupted and was infiltrated by polymorphonuclear leucocytes and mononuclear cells. *(H&E ×445)*

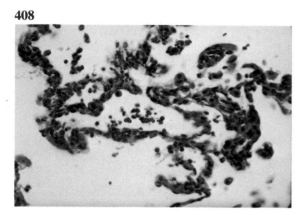

408 The interalveolar septa are infiltrated by polymorphonuclear leucocytes. *(H&E ×225)*

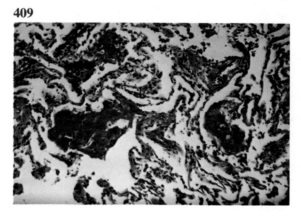

409 Alveoli containing leucocytes and erythrocytes in a protein rich exudate. *(H&E ×110)*

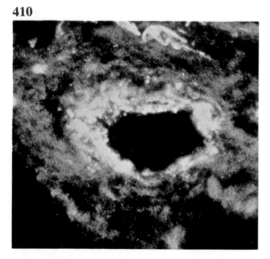

410 Prominent granular staining for C3 complement in a wall of a small vein. Immunofluorescence microscopy.

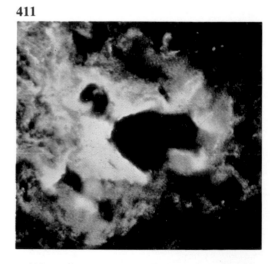

411 Behçet's disease. Staining for fibrinogen occurring in the wall of a small vein and adjacent perivascular tissue. Immunofluorescence microscopy.

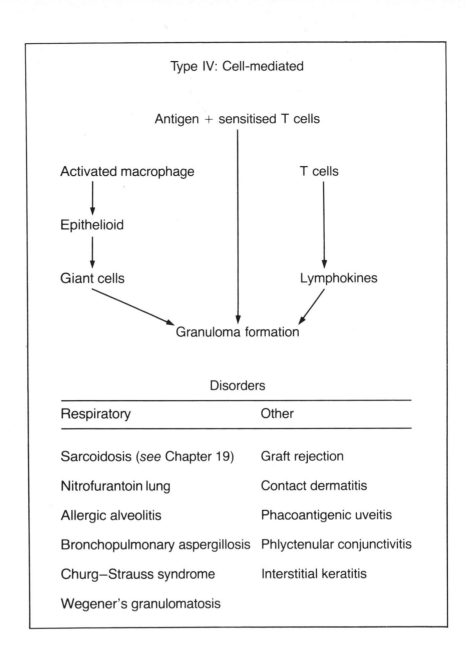

Type IV: Cell-mediated

Antigen + sensitised T cells

Activated macrophage   T cells

Epithelioid

Giant cells   Lymphokines

Granuloma formation

Disorders

Respiratory	Other
Sarcoidosis (*see* Chapter 19)	Graft rejection
Nitrofurantoin lung	Contact dermatitis
Allergic alveolitis	Phacoantigenic uveitis
Bronchopulmonary aspergillosis	Phlyctenular conjunctivitis
Churg–Strauss syndrome	Interstitial keratitis
Wegener's granulomatosis	

Allergic alveolitis (Hypersensitivity pneumonitis)

The repeated inhalation of various organic dusts (page 154) causes a hypersensitivity granulomatous pneumonitis, reflecting Type IV cell-mediated reactivity. There is also evidence of Type III reactivity with delayed-type skin tests and precipitating antibodies. Initially, repeated inhalation of the offending antigen leads to the production of circulating precipitating antibodies and to circulating immune complexes (Type III), but sufficient antigen invasion also leads to macrophage activation and to epithelioid cell granuloma formation (Type IV).

A frequent presentation is with breathlessness accompanied by dry cough, malaise, fever and limb pains. After heavy exposure symptoms develop about six hours later. Repeated exposure may result in irreversible lung fibrosis and chronic respiratory impairment.

Farmers' lung

412 Farmers' lung. The mouldy hay contrasts with the freshly stored. The principal organism responsible for farmers' lung is Micropolyspora faeni (85 per cent of cases) but the thermoactinomyces species is also important. When stored with a water content of about 40 per cent, hay, grain or other vegetable matter becomes heated as a result of the metabolism of rapidly multiplying thermophilic organisms. This is the best recognised example of extrinsic allergic alveolitis in the United Kingdom.

The presence of immunologically specific circulating precipitins points to the diagnosis. However, precipitins may be found in healthy exposed subjects with no lung disease, and may disappear quite quickly when exposure ceases in patients with irreversible lung damage.

412

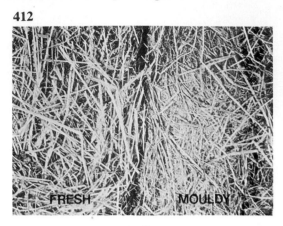

413

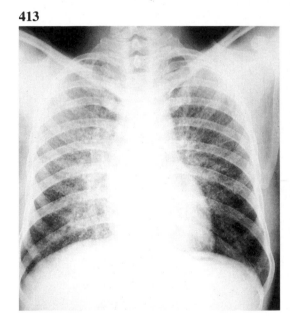

413 Acute farmers' lung. Fine nodular shadows are visible in the central two-thirds. Recurrent breathlessness, dry cough, influenza-like symptoms of malaise fever and limb pains occur at an interval of six hours after heavy exposure to mouldy hay. In mild attacks there may be no lung function abnormality. Severe attacks show a restrictive defect.

414

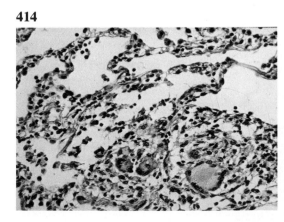

414 Farmers' lung. Focal granulomatous lesions together with a diffuse interstitial chronic inflammatory cell infiltrate of histiocytes and plasma cells are centred on the small bronchi. The non-caseating granulomas often contain characteristic clefts and doubly refractile foreign material of vegetable origin which distinguishes them from sarcoid lesions.

150

415

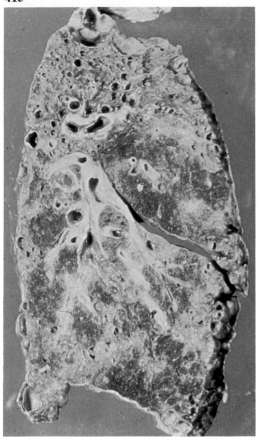

416a

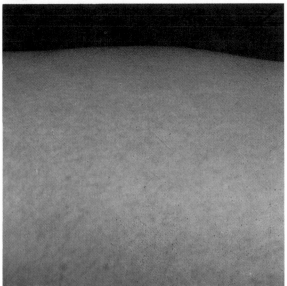

416a Farmers' lung. A late skin reaction (Type III) to M. faeni was observed six hours after an intradermal injection of 0.1 ml of test solution. Complement and IgG are classically involved and in most subjects specific precipitating antibody is present. Some late reactions may be mediated by IgE antibodies alone.

415 Chronic farmers' lung. This diffuse interstitial disease with fibrosis causes contraction and distortion of the alveoli to produce 'honeycombing' and cyst formation. The fibrotic changes are usually more prominent in the upper than in the lower zones. Cyanosis and finger clubbing may occur.

416b Bronchial challenge test to M. faeni (diagramatic). Late asthma (Type III) accompanied by moderate systemic symptoms maximal at 8 hours after challenge with M. faeni.

The other causes of extrinsic allergic alveolitis may produce similar bronchospasm on provocation testing.

The safety of bronchial provocation tests is often questioned. They should only be performed under medical supervision with facilities available to treat bronchospasm.

Skin and bronchial challenge tests are complementary in sorting out the specificity of antigens suspected to be the cause of extrinsic alveolitis.

416b

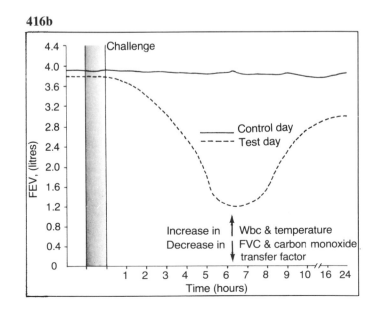

Avian protein hypersensitivity

Exposure to the dry dust of bird droppings, particularly the globulin fraction, and dust from the feathers of healthy birds, is responsible for the clinical features of bird fanciers' lung.

Pigeon fanciers whose exposure occurs intermittently when cleaning the loft often present with acute symptoms. Budgerigar fanciers are constantly exposed to birds kept indoors and more often present with chronic insidious lung disease.

Evidence of sensitisation to pigeon protein is found in 35 per cent of all pigeon breeders and it is likely that about 15 per cent of fanciers experience hypersensitivity reactions.

417

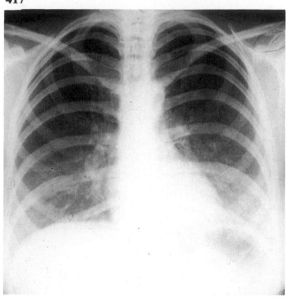

418

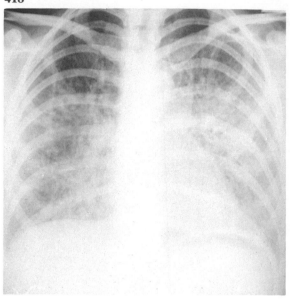

417 Acute extrinsic allergic alveolitis in a young budgerigar fancier with diffuse lower zone nodular shadowing. At this stage the patients' only symptoms were an irritating cough and a vague malaise.

418 Budgerigar fanciers' lung. Fine widely disseminated nodular shadows (ground glass) in association with severe dyspnoea, rigors and fever followed continuing heavy exposure to budgerigars. Lung volumes were greatly reduced. Fine inspiratory crackles were heard throughout both lung fields. (Seven weeks after **417**.)

419

419 Budgerigar fanciers' lung. Complete reversal of the symptoms and the radiographic shadowing occurred after removal from contact with the allergen. (Same patient as **417** and **418**.)

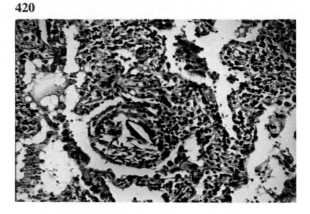

420 Acute pigeon fanciers' lung. Interstitial alveolar wall infiltrate of lymphocytes, plasma cells and foamy histiocytes and clefted granuloma are present. Unlike sarcoidosis the granulomas are not seen in the hilar lymph nodes and they resolve rapidly without hyalinisation. *(H&E ×100)*

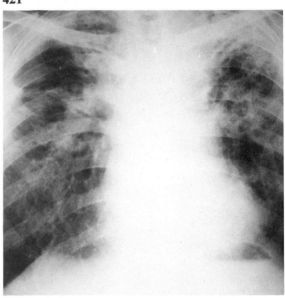

421 Chronic bird fanciers' lung. Upper lobe fibrosis and cavitation leading to a permanent severe ventilatory restriction and diffusion defect.

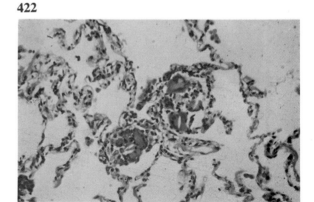

422 Chronic bird fanciers' lung with extensive fibrotic scarring and disorganisation of the normal alveolar structure and the development of honeycombing.

Table: Nature and sources of organic dust antigens in extrinsic allergic alveolitis.
(Probably IgE mediated obstructive airways disease)

Disease	Dust exposure	Nature of antigen to which precipitin shown
Farmers' lung	Mouldy overheated hay	Thermophilic actinomycetes Micropolyspora faeni Thermoactinomyces vulgaris
Fog-fever in cattle	Mouldy hay	Micropolyspora faeni
Bagassosis	Mouldy overheated sugar-cane bagasse	Mouldy bagasse Thermoactinomyces sacharii
Mushroom workers' lung	Mushroom compost dust	Thermophilic actinomycetes (see farmers' lung)
Maltworkers' lung	Mouldy barley or malt	Aspergillus fumigatus Aspergillus clavatus
Bird fanciers' lung	Pigeon and budgerigar droppings Wax coating feathers – 'pigeon bloom'	Avian serum protein antigens
Pituitary snufftakers' lung	Powder of porcine and bovine posterior-pituitary extract	Serum protein and pituitary antigens
Wheat weevil disease (Millers' lung)	Infested wheat flour	Sitophilus granarius
Maple strippers' lung	Maple bark	Cryptostroma (Coniosporium) corticale
Sequoiosis	Mouldy redwood sawdust	Aureobasidium (Pullularia) – pullulans – graphium
Suberosis	Oak bark, cork dust	Mouldy oak bark P. frequentans
Woodworkers' lung	Sawdusts of oak, cedar, etc.	Sawdust extracts
Cheese-washers' lung	Moulds on cheese	Penicillium casei
'New Guinea' lung	Mouldy thatch dust	Extracts of thatch
Smallpox-handlers' lung	Smallpox scabs	
Paprika splitters' lung	Mouldy paprika pods	Mucor stolonifer
Humidifier or forced-air-system lung	Fungal spores in air-conditioning ducts and in home humidifiers	T. candidus T. vulgaris Naegleria gruberi
Coptic lung	Cloth wrappings of mummies	
Poultry handlers' lung	Poultry feathers and products	Turkey and chicken proteins
Coffee and tea growers' disease	Green coffee bean Tea fluff	

Wegener's granulomatosis

Wegener's granulomatosis is a granulomatous angiitis in particular involving the nasal mucosa, trachea, larynx, lungs, and kidney. Onset is usually insidious and occurs during the fourth or fifth decade. The course is usually relentless and progressive resulting in intractable sinusitis, nodular pulmonary lesions and terminal renal involvement. Biopsy shows ulcerating granulomatous angiitis, in which pulmonary vessels are especially involved. This suggests Type IV reactivity, but evidence of immune complexes and renal disease also suggest Type III injury. The disease may be localised to the lungs or widely disseminated (see Table on page 129).

423

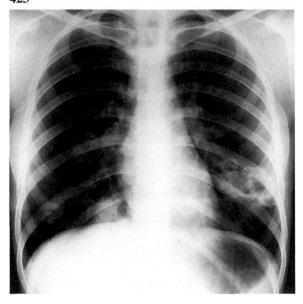

423 Localised Wegener's granulomatosis. Multiple bilateral nodular lesions are present in the lower zones.

424

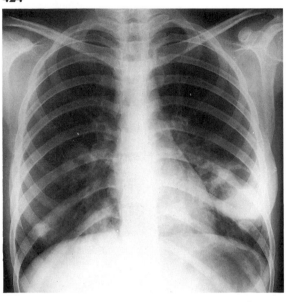

424 Localised Wegener's granulomatosis. One month later cavitation in the left lung has increased as a consequence of local vasculitis and gangrene.

425

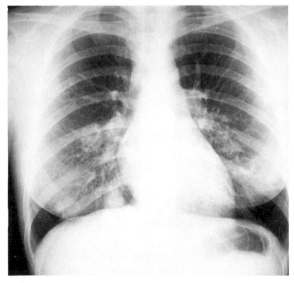

425 Localised Wegener's granulomatosis. After two months' immunosuppressive therapy the cavitating lesions have partially healed.

426a and b Generalised Wegener's granulomatosis. Upper respiratory tract lesions destroy nasal cartilage, and produce a saddle nose deformity. Nasal biopsy is worthwhile.

426 a
426 b

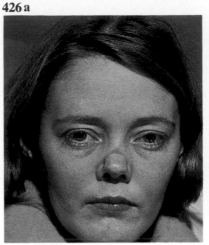

427

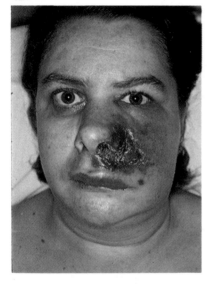

428

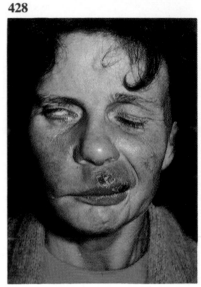

428 Generalised Wegener's granulomatosis. This patient developed a right seventh cranial nerve palsy, vasculitis of the upper lip and pulmonary cavitation. The central nervous system and kidney may both be involved by widespread vasculitis. There is also vasculitis of the upper lip.

427 Pyoderma gangrenosum can occur. This florid ulceration extended into the nostrils. Immunosuppressive drug treatment produced rapid healing.

429

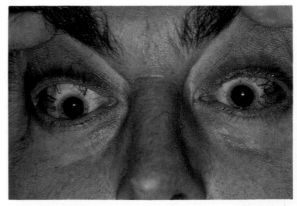

429 Bilateral scleritis. There was also iridocyclitis, retinal vasculitis and minimal conjunctivitis.

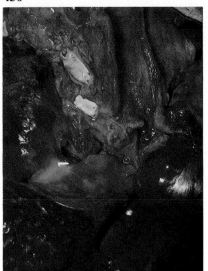

431

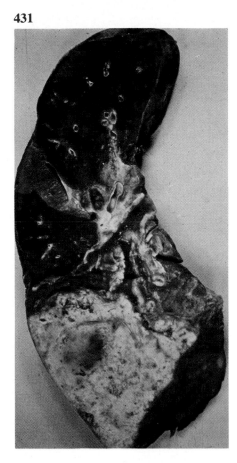

430 Wegener's granulomatosis. Haemorrhagic ulceration of the trachea and bronchi. The cut surface of the lower lobe is haemorrhagic from a terminal infarction.

431 Wegener's granulomatosis. A large creamy yellow infarcted lesion involves most of the lower lobe. Necrosis is followed by cavitation.

432

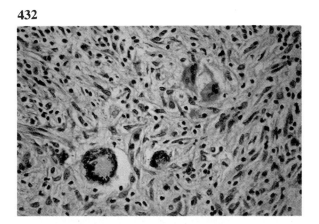

433

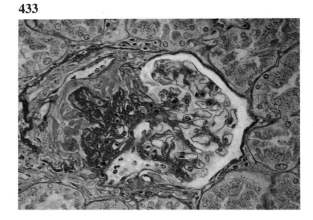

432 Wegener's granulomatosis. Cellular infiltrate and necrotising granulomas situated in relationship to the bronchi and at the periphery of infarcted lesions.

433 Wegener's granulomatosis. Glomerular involvement with necrosis and angiitis in the capillary tuft and eosinophilic fibrinoid degeneration are characteristic histological findings.

Polyarteritis nodosa

Polyarteritis nodosa (PAN) is a collagen disease characterised by inflammatory and necrotising lesions in all three layers of small arteries and arterioles leading to aneurysm, thrombosis and infarction. Men are affected four times more frequently than women. Clinical features are a rapid deterioration with unexplained fever, weightloss, a high sedimentation rate, hypertension and glomerulonephritis, neurological involvement, arthritis and abdominal pain. Lung involvement presents with cough, haemoptysis, pneumonia and asthmatic symptoms. A very high blood eosinophilia points to the diagnosis which may be confirmed by finding arthritic lesions in skin or muscle biopsy or visceral aneurysm on angiography. Apart from a strong association with hepatitis B antigen, only minor immunological abnormalities are found in PAN.

The Churg–Strauss syndrome of eosinophilic granulomatosis is delineated as a variant of polyarteritis nodosa because of asthma, granuloma formation and generalised vasculitis. Visceral angiography reveals aneurysms. Raised IgE levels, possible immune complex and cell-mediated granulomas all indicate Type I, II and IV lung injury (see Table on page 129).

434

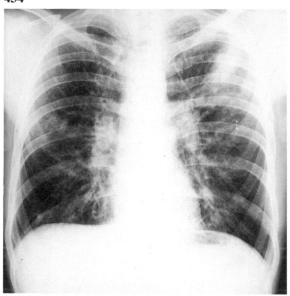

434 Polyarteritis nodosa with pulmonary infiltration. Pleurisy with pleural effusion may be present.

435

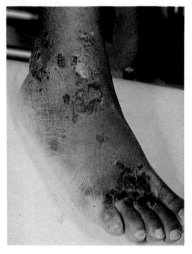

435 Mononeuritis with vasculitis in polyarteritis nodosa.

436

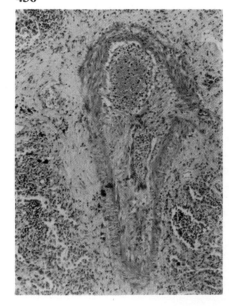

436 Polyarteritis nodosa. Arteritis usually begins in the media and extends to the outer coats of the arterial wall; necrosis, inflammatory cell infiltration and eventual healing with fibrosis then follow. The vessel wall is partially destroyed and the lumen occluded by thrombosis.

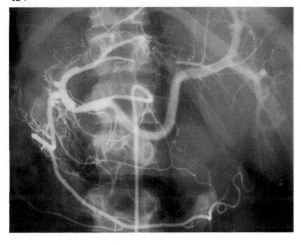

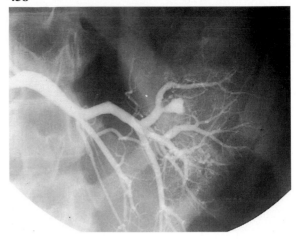

437 Visceral angiography. Aneurysms are demonstrated in the splenic artery and left hepatic artery.

438 Visceral angiography. Magnified renal arteriogram demonstrating aneurysms of the renal artery.

Table: Causes of necrotising angiitis.

Polyarteritis nodosa
  – Classical
  – HBsAg associated in 20 per cent

Churg–Strauss eosinophilic granulomatosis

Wegener's granulomatosis (*see* page 155)

Systemic lupus erythematosus (*see* page 145)

Behçet's syndrome (*see* page 146)

Henoch–Schonlein purpura

Arteritis
  – Hypersensitivity angiitis

  – Giant-cell temporal

  – Takayasu's pulseless aortic

  – Retinal vasculitis

  – Rheumatoid arthritis (*see* page 143)

  – Rheumatic fever

Lymphomatoid granulomatosis

This form of angiitis and granulomatosis, first described in 1972, closely resembles localised Wegener's granulomatosis and usually presents in middle age, slightly more often in males, with fever, cough and dyspnoea. Extrapulmonary manifestations include a raised erythematous skin rash resembling erythema nodosum but on the trunk, skin nodules, central nervous system involvement with cranial nerve palsies, peripheral neuropathy, hepatosplenomegaly or peripheral lymphadenopathy. Most patients die within three years and 12 per cent develop malignant lymphoma.

440

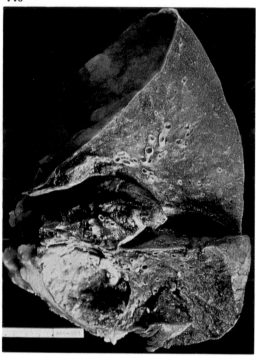

440 Lymphomatoid granulomatosis. Extensive necrosis with cavitation of a large nodular lesion in the left lung.

Angioimmunoblastic lymphadenopathy

442 Angioimmunoblastic lymphadenopathy. The normal lymph node architecture is replaced by a mixed cellular proliferation of immunoblasts and plasma cells which also may infiltrate the lung. Patients present with fever, lymphadenopathy, anaemia, polyclonal hyper-gamma-globulinaemia and pulmonary changes reminiscent of Hodgkin's disease. *(H&E ×40)*

439

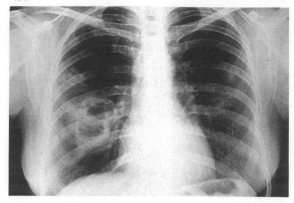

439 Lymphomatoid granulomatosis. Bilateral opacities and cavitation in the right mid-zone. The main radiographic features are of multiple bilateral opacities resembling metastases and the absence of hilar adenopathy.

441

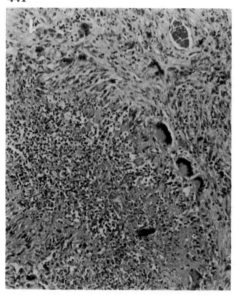

441 Lymphomatoid granulomatosis. A highly cellular atypical lymphoreticular infiltrate, rich in mitosis, which often invades or destroys blood vessels.

442

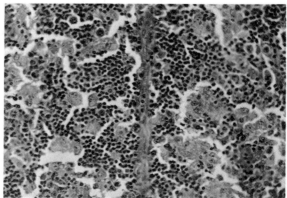

18 Interstitial lung disease

The description 'interstitial lung disease' is often used to refer to a wide range of different processes which involve the peripheral gas exchanging areas of the lung. This results in functional impairment of gas transfer and a restrictive defect of ventilation. Implied is that the disease process involves the acini and associated supporting tissue.

Acute alveolitis follows in the wake of acinar injury involving Type I and Type II epithelial cells in the alveolar walls. If the injury should persist, the surrounding connective tissue becomes involved, collagenases disrupt collagen and lung tissue is destroyed. The end stage histology is of non-specific irreversible pulmonary fibrosis with few helpful diagnostic features. These changes are best described as diffuse pulmonary alveolar or acinar fibrosis. A classification is outlined (*see* tables).

Table: Classification of interstitial lung disease.

Known aetiology	Unknown aetiology

Dusts
  – Organic (*see* page 154)
  – Inorganic (*see* page 162)
	Necrotising angiitis (*see* page 159)
	
	Collagen disorders
	  – Rheumatoid arthritis
	  – Progressive systemic sclerosis
	  – Sjogren's syndrome
	  – Ankylosing spondylitis (*see* page 176)

Fumes (*see* page 171)	

Drugs (*see* page 171)	Inherited disorders
	  – Tuberous sclerosis
	  – Neurofibromatosis

Infections
  – Schistosoma mansoni
	Miscellaneous
	  – Sarcoidosis (*see* Chapter 19)
	  – Goodpasture's syndrome (*see* page 142)
	  – Eosinophilic granuloma
	  – Idiopathic haemosiderosis
	  – Amyloidosis
	  – Veno-occlusive disease
	  – Idiopathic pulmonary fibrosis
	  – Lymphangioleiomyomatosis

Pulmonary oedema	
Uraemia	
Irradiation	

Table: Causes of occupational interstitial lung disease.

Inorganic dust	Industrial hazard
Aluminium	Grinding
Asbestos	Mining Fireproofing Lagging Dock workers
Beryllium } Cadmium }	Alloys Electronics Nuclear workers
Coal ⎤ Diatomaceous earth ⎥ Graphite ⎬ Kaolin ⎥ Mica ⎦	Mining Processing Polishing
Iron oxide (Siderosis)	Welding
Silica	Mining and manufacturing Drilling, blasting Foundry and glass workers
Talc	Ceramics and cosmetics
Titanium	Paint

Pneumoconiosis

The literal meaning of pneumoconiosis is 'dusty lung'. An acceptable definition is 'the presence of inhaled dust in the lungs and their non-neoplastic tissue reaction to it'.

Inhaled dust particles are a hazard in certain occupations, because if inhaled they may reach the terminal bronchioles and alveoli to initiate destructive reactions and fibrosis.

The particle size is important. Particles in the range $0.5\,\mu$m to $5\,\mu$m may reach the alveoli, especially in the mid zone of the lungs. Larger particles impact in the proximal airways and are removed by muco-ciliary clearance. Particles less than $0.5\,\mu$m behave like a gas and seldom settle in the lungs.

The inhaled non-reactive dusts of tin, iron, barium and antimony may produce extensive pulmonary shadowing with little if any functional impairment.

Coal dust, kaolin and diatomaceous earth may cause moderate functional changes, while severe functional impairment may be caused by inhaling the highly fibrogenic dusts of silica, talc and asbestos.

The clinical significance of dust exposure can be difficult to evaluate because of the overwhelming effect of cigarette smoking. In some studies the effect of cigarette smoking on the fall of FEV_1 was up to five times greater than any effect caused by dust.

Coal-miners' pneumoconiosis

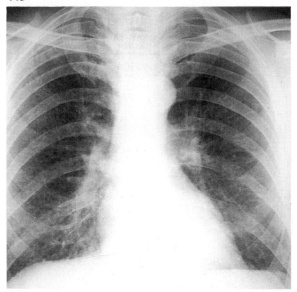

443   **Simple coal-miners' pneumoconiosis.** Minute opacities are diffusely scattered throughout both lung fields, providing a crude measure of excessive exposure. Early pneumoconiosis is essentially a focal disorder and may produce little physiological disturbance.

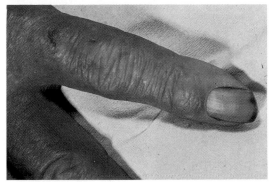

444   **Coal-miners' scars** pigmented by coal dust, give a clue to the cause of underlying lung disease. Advanced pneumoconiosis is a serious disorder with a poor prognosis. The more prevalent early stages of either coal-miners' pneumoconiosis or silicosis are associated with little physiological impairment.

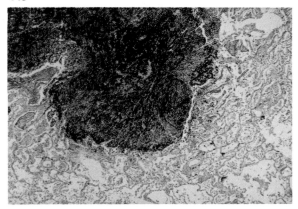

445   **Atherosilicotic nodule.** These arise in the walls of alveoli and respiratory bronchioles and lead to destruction of the bronchiolar muscle and formation of dense collagen which obliterates the bronchiolar lumen and vascular channels. Unlike the true silicotic nodule, the collagen is arranged in an irregular pattern. The process may progress to centrilobular emphysema and fibrosis.

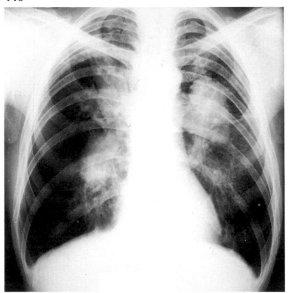

446   **Progressive massive fibrosis** describes the development of nodular lesions in the lungs larger than 1 cm in diameter. Single or multiple large fibrotic masses, irregular in shape, are present in the upper and right middle lobes. Cavitation and emphysematous changes may supervene.

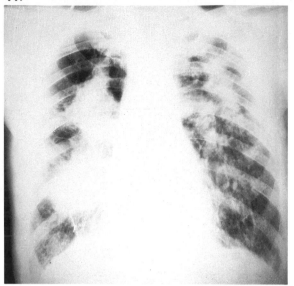

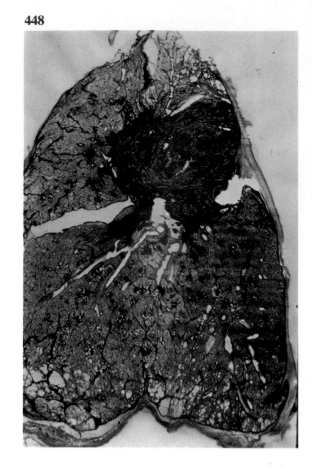

447 Progressive massive fibrosis. Large progressive lesions with considerable distortion of the right lung. Advanced coal-workers' pneumoconiosis may terminate in cor pulmonale.

448 Simple coal dust foci and basal emphysema shown in thick whole lung section together with a large solid anthrocotic area of progressive massive fibrosis.

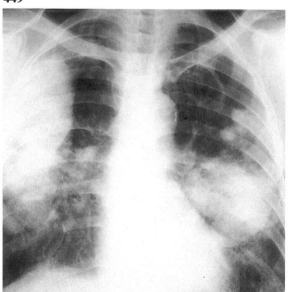

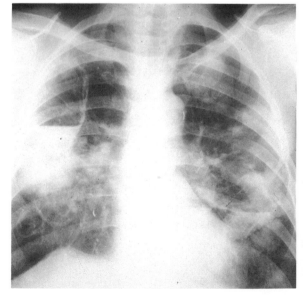

449 Progressive massive fibrosis (PMF). The usual discrete xray shadows seen in silicosis and coalworkers' pneumoconiosis may coalesce to form large masses of collagen, especialy in those with rheumatoid arthritis. This example shows unusually large opacities.

450 Progressive massive fibrosis (PMF). The centre of the mass may become necrotic and liquify. Copious black sputum (melanoptysis) was expectorated leaving these partially fluid-filled cavities (same patient as **449**).

451

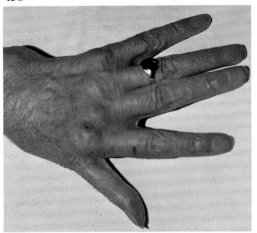

451 Coal-miners' tattoo and rheumatoid arthritis indicating rheumatoid pneumoconiosis. Vasculitis on the knuckle of the first finger is also evident.

452

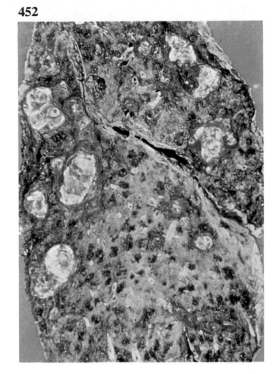

452 Caplan's lesions (rheumatoid pneumoconiosis). The lung section showing rheumatoid nodules. These lesions may precede or follow clinical evidence of rheumatoid arthritis. Cellular and necrotising reactions occur at the periphery of silicotic nodules. Concentric calcification is common.

Silicosis

Silicosis is caused by inhalation of fine free crystalline silica dioxide dust or quartz particles. Silicosis occurs in slate and granite quarrying, refractory and foundry work, and in the glass and pottery industries.

453

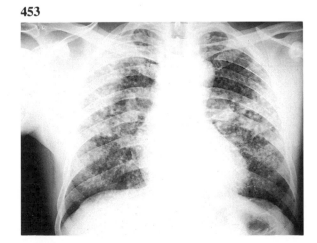

453 Simple silicosis showing diffuse widespread nodular lesions most marked in the mid-zone. The nodules increase in size and coalesce as the disease progresses. Disability is caused by restriction in lung volumes. At a late stage eggshell calcification of the hilar glands may occur. Simple silicosis describes the xray appearance of fine nodulation with no conglomerate nodule greater than 1 cm in diameter.

454

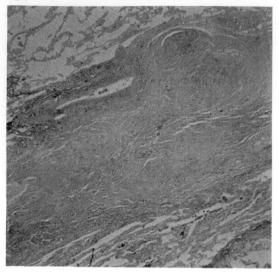

454 Silicotic nodules arise in the alveolar walls. Collagen deposited concentrically causes obliterative bronchiolitis. Silica, if present, is found peripherally. In contrast to the lesions in coal pneumoconiosis, the silicotic lesions are proliferative with an excess of collagen but little silica dust. The inhaled free crystalline silica or silicon dioxide particles are ingested by macrophages and probably converted to salicic acid. The macrophages respond to the 'irritation' by liberating lysosomal enzymes which, it is believed, play an important part in pathogenesis.

The amount of dust present in the lung is small relative to the severity of the fibrosis produced.

The fibrosis may extend despite cessation of dust exposure. Isolated nodules may coalesce to form large conglomerates of fibrous tissue, situated especially in the upper parts of the lungs. The condition is then known as complicated pneumoconiosis or progressive massive fibrosis.

456 Silicotuberculosis. A thick-walled tuberculous apical cavity and extensive pulmonary fibrosis in a foundry-fettler.

Silica and silicon dioxide react synergistically with mycobacteria; their growth rate on culture media is accelerated and host immunity to mycobacteria is reduced. Atypical mycobacteria, usually M. kansasii are frequent pathogens.

Asbestos exposure

Asbestos is a mixture of the silicates of iron, magnesium, nickel, calcium and aluminium. The main types of asbestos are chrysotile (which accounts for about 90 per cent of the world production), crocidolite or blue asbestos, amosite and anthophyllite. The needle-shaped asbestos particles are from $20\,\mu$m to $100\,\mu$m long and less than $3\,\mu$m thick. Inhaled fibres impact in the lower bronchi and alveoli, whence they may reach the pleura, diaphragm or even peritoneum.

455

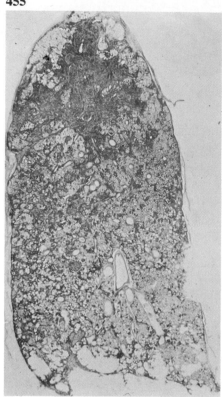

455 Silicosis in a slate worker. This whole lung section shows multiple greyish nodules and massive fibrosis in the upper lobe.

456

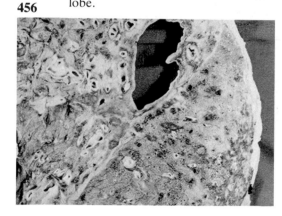

Asbestos-induced disorders are:
1 Diffuse interstitial fibrosis (asbestosis)
2 Pleural fibrosis and plaque formation
3 Malignant mesothelioma of the pleura or peritoneum
4 An increased incidence of bronchial carcinoma

Workers in many industries are exposed to raw asbestos with potential hazard to health.

A code of practice for the safe handling of this valuable mineral is enforced by law in the United Kingdom and many other countries. There is no effective treatment for asbestosis other than prevention.

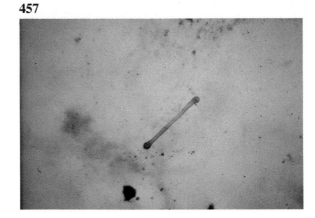

457 Asbestos bodies in sputum. The asbestos fibre becomes coated with a film of proteinaceous material which is thickened over the sharp ends giving a bulbous appearance.

458

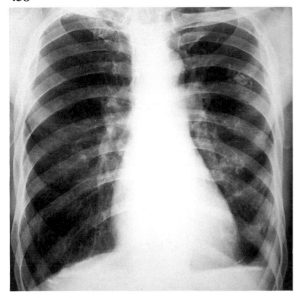

459

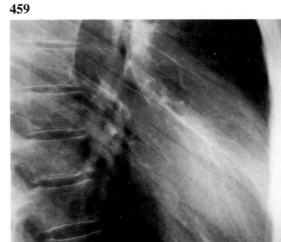

458 and 459 Diaphragmatic calcification. Asbestos pleural plaques calcify bilaterally on the diaphragm and lower half of the parietal pleura. This dock worker had unloaded raw asbestos.

460

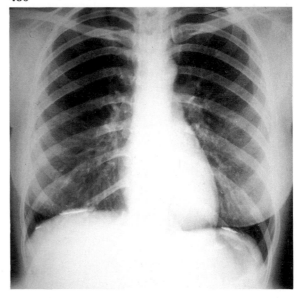

460 Pleural plaques. This dock worker's daughter was exposed to asbestos from her father's clothing.

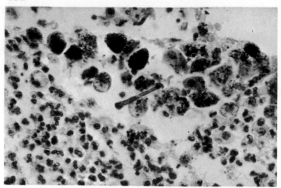

461

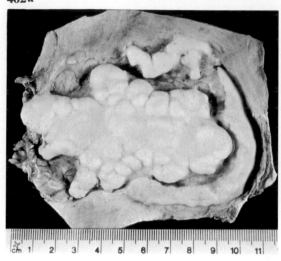

462a

461 Asbestos bodies in the lung gradually shrink and eventually leave a collection of dark granules of iron oxide.

462a and b Parietal pleural plaques. Pleural plaques are localised thickenings of the parietal pleura with dense hyaline collagen which may calcify. The radiographic detection depends upon the size and degree of calcification.

462a was visible on chest xray as a large calcified diaphragmatic plaque but none of the plaques on **462b** was visible.

Plaques are usually bilateral and occur most commonly over the middle and lower posterolateral chest wall and central portion of the diaphragm. Only 15 per cent are detectable in life. They do not significantly interfere with lung function unless the pleura is extensively thickened.

462b

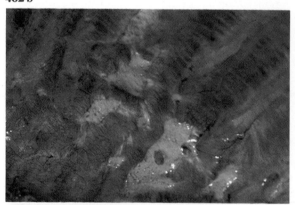

463

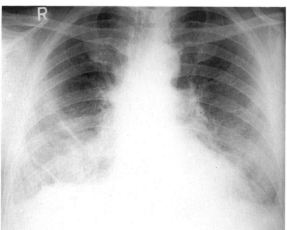

464

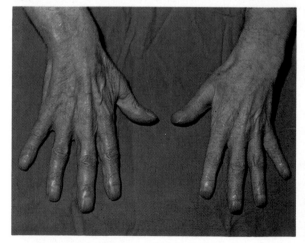

463 Lung fibrosis (asbestosis) after ten years of heavy asbestos exposure in a pipe lagger. Lower zone streaky fibrosis obscures the diaphragms and gives the cardiac silhouette a 'shaggy' appearance. Some 35 per cent of patients with asbestosis develop bronchial carcinoma, the risk being further increased if tobacco is smoked.

464 Cyanosis and finger clubbing signify a late stage of asbestosis. The commonest complaint is of exercise-induced breathlessness. Auscultation of the chest usually reveals loud inspiratory crackles best heard at the lung bases.

Finger clubbing is present in one-third. Asbestosis causes a restrictive respiratory defect and shortens life: 20 per cent will die from respiratory failure.

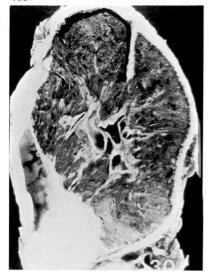

 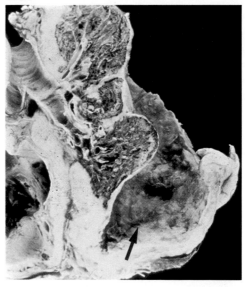

465a Diffuse pulmonary (asbestosis) and pleural disease usually occur together after prolonged and substantial asbestos exposure. The lung is encased by thickened pleura and the lung structure distorted by fibrosis. Lung function tests showed greatly reduced lung volumes (left lung section).

466

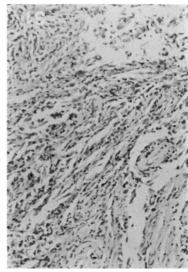

465b Pleural mesothelioma and diffuse pleural disease. The mesothelioma (arrowed) is infiltrating the pleura and displacing adjacent lung. Typically there is a latent period of 20 years or more between first exposure to asbestos and the development of mesothelioma. Present evidence suggests that any heavy asbestos exposure but particularly to crocidolite (blue) may cause a malignant mesothelioma.

466 Mesothelioma. A uniform 'spindle cell' or sarcomatous appearance is most usual on histology. In some, the appearance mimics adenocarcinoma and confident diagnosis is only established at necropsy.

467

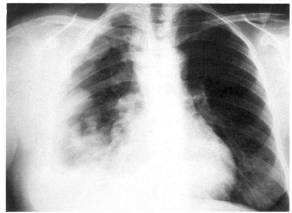

468

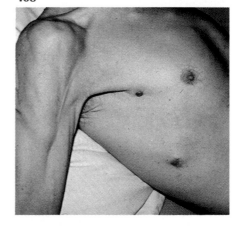

467 Pleural mesothelioma. Irregular protuberant pleural opacities give rise to blood-stained effusions. Symptoms are of breathlessness, weightloss and pleurisy.

468 Mesothelial tumours spread locally and grow along needle and incision tracks.

Benign non-fibrotic pneumoconioses

These are recognised by the presence of multiple small dense opacities on chest xray caused by perivascular collections of dust with increase in reticulin fibres but no collagen. Lung function is unchanged and there are no symptoms. The dusts responsible include iron dust (siderosis) from mining and processing iron ore and steel, oxides of iron from welding, barium sulphate (baritosis), antimony and chromate dusts.

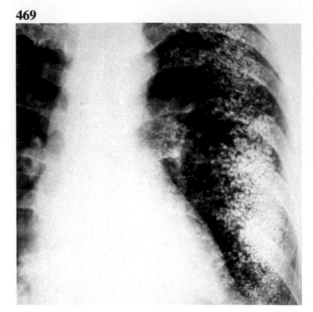

469

469   Stannosis. This is caused by the inhalation of tin dust produced by mining, or tin oxide fumes from smelting.

Small radiodense opacities are scattered throughout the lung. Inhalation of inert tin dust has no known effect upon lung function or health and is another cause of benign non-fibrotic pneumoconiosis.

Byssinosis

470   Byssinosis. This occurs in workers exposed to the inhalation of dusts from raw cotton, flax or hemp. After prolonged exposure the worker becomes breathless at work on re-exposure. This 'Monday feeling' may improve as the week progresses but eventually constant symptoms of cough, sputum production and breathlessness are indistinguishable from chronic bronchitis.

The raw cotton may be directly antigenic or alternatively the symptoms may be caused by the inhalation of large numbers of Gram-negative bacteria contained in the cotton. There are no specific xray features. The pathological changes are mostly non-specific with features similar to those found in chronic bronchitis. However, fibrosis related mainly to the bronchi and emphysematous changes present adjacent to dust foci are described. The pathogenesis is not understood, nor is the curious pattern of respiratory reaction which is neither due solely to irritation or allergy.

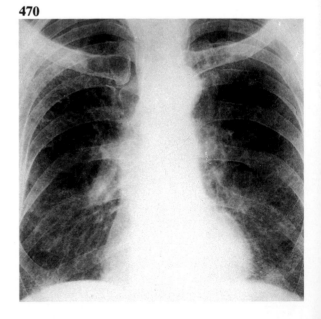

470

Beryllium disease

Beryllium disease (berylliosis) affects those engaged in extracting the metal from the ores or those who handle beryllium compounds. Individual susceptibility is an important factor, because only two per cent of those at risk develop berylliosis. Exposure may result in an acute reaction with pulmonary oedema and pneumonia or a chronic granulomatous reaction.

471

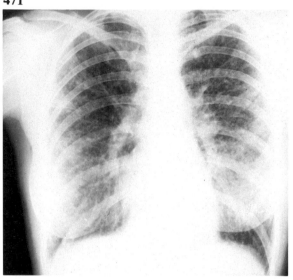

471 Chronic beryllium disease with pulmonary infiltration resembling sarcoidosis.

472

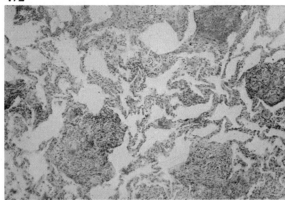

472 Beryllium disease showing sarcoid granulomas with fibrosis. A history of exposure to beryllium, a negative Kveim test, normal serum angiotensin-converting enzyme and the presence of beryllium in the tissue or urine confirm the diagnosis.

Table: Fumes causing interstitial lung disease.

Exposure	Vapour inhaled
Swimming pools	Chlorine gas
Ore-smelting	Sulphur dioxide
Nose drops	Oil
Vineyard spray	Bordeaux mixture of copper sulphate and lime
Insecticides	Pyrethrum

(*See* page 138 for inhalants causing occupational asthma)

Table: Causes of drug-induced chronic interstitial lung disease.

Busulphan	Diphenylhydantoin
Bleomycin	Gold salts
Chlorambucil	Nitrofurantoin
Cyclophosphamide	Paraquat
Methotrexate	Penicillin
Nitrosoureas	Pentolinium
Procarbazine	Sulphonamides
Vincristine	

Drugs produce a variety of adverse effects in the lungs with involvement of the lung parenchyma, the airways or the pulmonary vasculature (*see* Table on page 171).

473

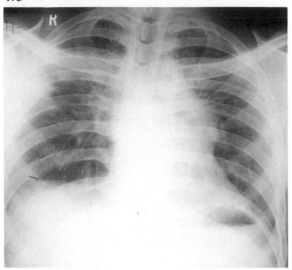

474

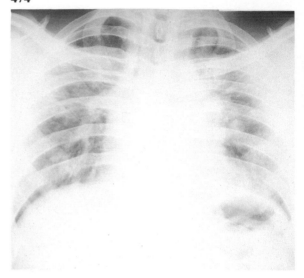

473 Cyclophosphamide lung. This diffuse pneumonitis developed in a 17-year-old boy who received the drug for three years as treatment for glomerulonephritis.

474 Cyclophosphamide lung. Widespread and progressive fibrosis with severe restriction in lung volumes three years after the drug was discontinued.

475a

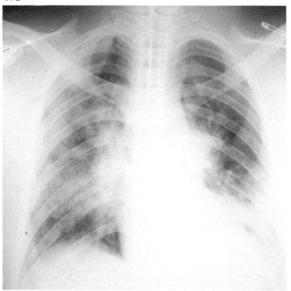

475b

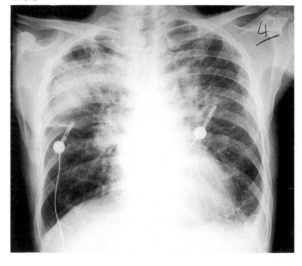

475a Non-cardiogenic pulmonary oedema. Severe pulmonary oedema as a result of heroin abuse. During the course of the illness this patient developed the acute adult respiratory distress syndrome and required assisted ventilation.

475b Chronic pulmonary oedema may produce confusing diffuse pulmonary shadowing. This right upper lobe consolidation was mistakenly thought to be caused by a bronchial carcinoma until complete clearing occurred with diuretics.

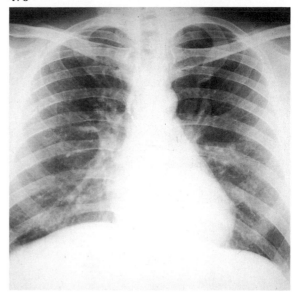

476

476 Diffuse interstitial fibrosis caused by schisto-somiasis (bilharziasis). A persistent progressive diffuse interstitial fibrosis follows infection with Schistosoma mansoni. The eggs lodge in pulmonary arterioles and the liberated schistoma glycoprotein antigen sets up a T-cell mediated immune response with perivascular granuloma formation involving the alveolar inter-stitium.

477

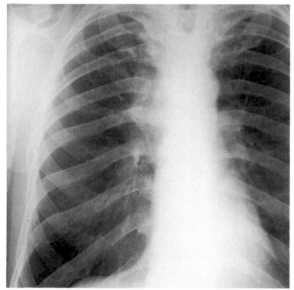

478

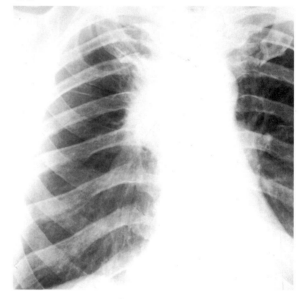

477 Radiation changes in the lung. PA film showing a right malignant paratracheal mass. The patient pre-sented with superior vena caval obstruction which resolved with radiotherapy.

478 Radiation changes in the lung. Twelve months after radiotherapy. Fibrosis developed after a latent period. The right upper zone is avascular with streaky line shadows (same as **477**).

Progressive systemic sclerosis

In systemic sclerosis increased production of mature collagen is followed by changes in the skin and involved organs. Typically, scleroderma, calcinosis, telangiectasia and Raynaud's phenomenon occur.

479

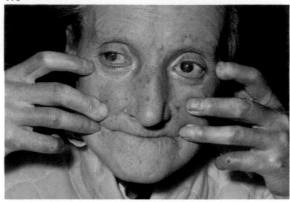

479 Systemic sclerosis. The skin is thickened around the mouth and hands, the latter also showing acrocyanosis caused by Raynaud's erosion of the terminal phalanges.

480

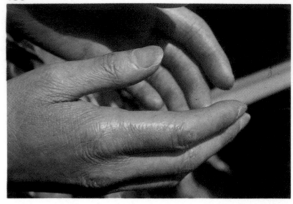

480 Systemic sclerosis. The hands are stiff and shiny.

481

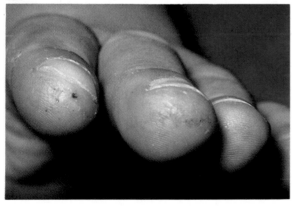

481 Systemic sclerosis. There is calcinosis of the fingertips.

482

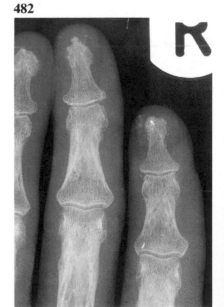

482 Radiograph of the fingertip in systemic sclerosis showing speckled calcification in the soft tissue.

483

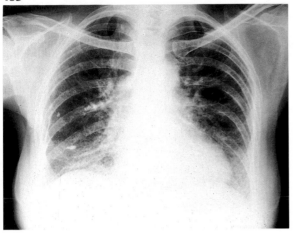

484

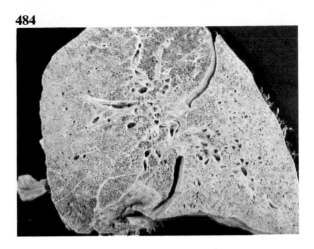

484 Lung in systemic sclerosis showing diffuse interstitial fibrosis and honeycombing (barium preparation).

483 Systemic sclerosis causes interstitial fibrosis and streaky or honeycomb changes particularly in the middle and lower zones. These lead to progressive dyspnoea, hypoxaemia, and ventilation-perfusion imbalance. Measurement of lung volumes shows a destructive defect and gas transfer is reduced.

485

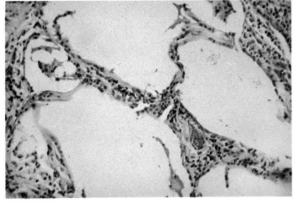

486

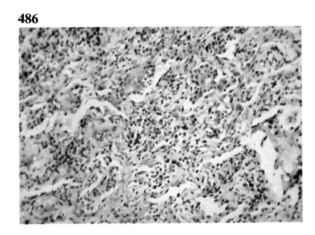

485 Progressive systemic sclerosis. Prominent alveolar capillaries and thickened acellular alveolar walls are characteristic of the earlier stages. *(H&E ×140)*

486 Progressive systemic sclerosis with intra-alveolar and interstitial fibrosis, disruption of alveolar walls and lymphocytic infiltration.

487

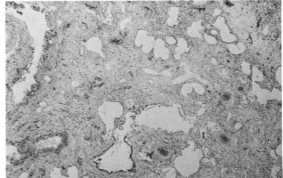

487 Progressive systemic sclerosis. Advanced fibrosis and honeycombing with collagenous thickening of the alveolar walls obliterating the normal architecture.

Sjögren's syndrome

Sjögren's syndrome occurs predominantly in menopausal women, presenting with keratoconjunctivitis sicca, dry mouth, parotid-gland enlargement, arthritis and chronic interstitial lung disease. It has features of an autoimmune disorder with circulating autoantibodies, plasma-cell infiltration of various tissues, and the co-existence of other autoimmune disorders including rheumatoid arthritis. The primary sicca syndrome without arthritis is associated with HLA-DRW3, and the rheumatoid arthritis-associated secondary sicca syndrome is HLA-DRW4-associated, indicating two different patterns of the disorder. Circulating immune complexes, a defective clearance rate of the reticuloendothelial system, and a high incidence of lymphomas are other features.

488

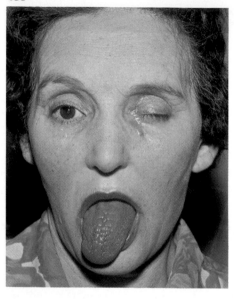

488 Dry fissured tongue and kerato-conjunctivitis sicca. Because of the very dry eyes this patient developed left corneal ulceration which required tarsorrhaphy.

489

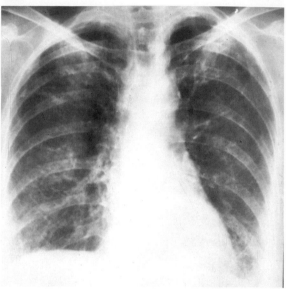

489 Pulmonary fibrosis in Sjögren's syndrome. The alveolar walls are infiltrated by mononuclear cells and become fibrosed. Recurrent pneumonia is common.

Ankylosing spondylitis

Ankylosing spondylitis results in increasing fixation of the thoracic cage and a restrictive pattern on lung function tests.

Lung fibrosis and apical cavitation are also described.

490 Ankylosing spondylitis causes rigidity of the thoracic cage, partly compensated by diaphragmatic movement. The anterior chest is flattened and the back immobile.

491 Ankylosing spondylitis. The anterior spinal ligaments of the thoracic spine become calcified ('bamboo' appearance).

490

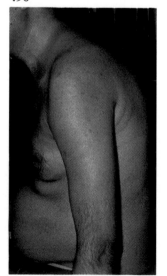

491

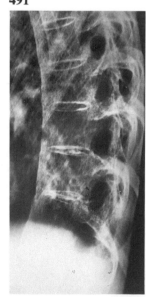

Tuberous sclerosis

This is an autosomal dominant inherited disorder originally described in 1880 as a classical clinical triad of mental retardation, epileptic seizures and dermal angiofibromas (adenoma sebaceum). Hamartomatous proliferative lesions occur causing parenchymal destructive and diffuse cystic disease generally throughout the body.

Pneumothorax, airflow obstruction with hypoxia and pulmonary cystic disease with focal nodular adenomatoid proliferation are described.

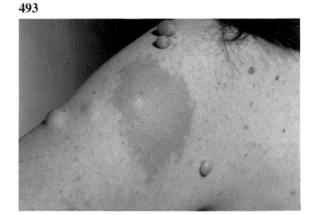

492   Tuberous sclerosis. Malar and nasal adenoma sebaceum in a mentally retarded patient. Similar nodules were present around the fingernails (sub-ungual fibromas). A diffuse non-specific reticulo-nodular pattern was seen on chest xray (not shown).

Neurofibromatosis (Von Recklinghausen's disease)

This is an inherited autosomal dominant disorder. Multiple neurofibromas may disfigure the skin and disrupt the nervous system. A number of skeletal anomalies may distort the skeleton.

Phaeochromocytoma is an infrequent accompaniment of the disease. In about five per cent of cases a neurofibroma will develop sarcomatous change.

493   Dermal neurofibromatosis together with irregular skin pigmentation; the characteristic 'cafe-au-lait' spots.

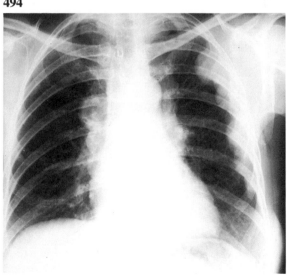

494   Neurofibromatosis. Posteroanterior chest xray showing multiple thoracic neurofibromas. Two other pulmonary manifestations are described; either honey-comb lung with non-specific clinical and functional changes or a fibrosing alveolitis-like picture.

Histiocytosis X (eosinophilic granuloma)

There is a progressive proliferation of histiocytes and infiltration of eosinophils in the lungs, bone and pituitary fossa. The lungs show granulomas, fibrosis and honeycombing. It occurs in adults between 20 and 40 years of age, presenting with interstitial lung disease, spontaneous pneumothorax, diabetes insipidus and bone involvement. The T cells lack H2 receptor sites, indicating a deficiency of suppressor T cells; and circulating lymphocytes are cytotoxic to cultured human fibroblasts.

495

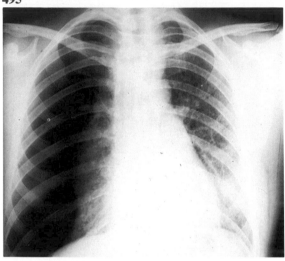

495 Histiocytosis X in a young male with diabetes insipidus. The chest xray shows miliary mottling involving the left lung. His chest disease was complicated by a right spontaneous pneumothorax.

497

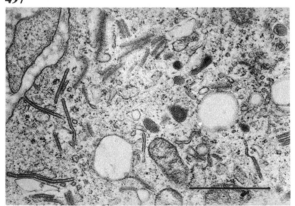

497 Histiocytosis X cell. The presence of the 'tennis-racquet'-shaped cytoplasmic organelles is diagnostic. (EM ×40,000)

498 Honeycomb lung caused by eosinophilic granuloma. The bullae ruptured and caused a fatal tension pneumothorax.

The disease is recognised in three forms:

1 Letterer–Siwe disease A fatal disorder of infants with splenomegaly, lymphadenopathy and cystic granulomatous lesions in the lungs.

2 Hand–Schüller–Christian disease Xanthomatous deposits cause miliary radiographic lung shadows, diabetes insipidus and bone cysts.

3 Eosinophilic granuloma Bone cysts are common. Pulmonary infiltration leads to fibrosis and bulla formation in about one-quarter of patients.

496

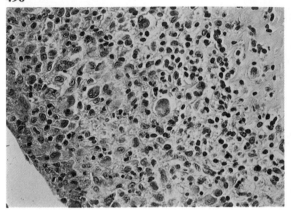

496 Histiocytosis X. Bronchial biopsy. Histiocytic cells, lymphocytes and plasma cells are present in this cavitating granuloma. (H&E ×280)

498

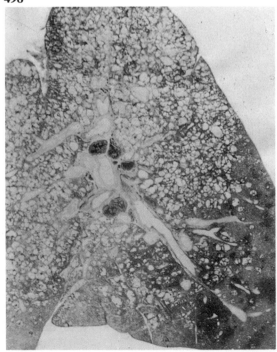

Idiopathic pulmonary haemosiderosis

Idiopathic pulmonary haemosiderosis (IPH) is a combination of interstitial fibrosis, haemosiderosis and recurrent intrapulmonary haemorrhage. The differential diagnosis includes Goodpasture's syndrome and systemic lupus erythematosus. However, the renal disease of Goodpasture's syndrome and the serum antibodies and other immunological features of SLE are absent. IPH is most common in young children who may develop anaemia in excess of the apparent blood loss from haemoptysis. Repeated attacks may lead to pulmonary hypertension, hepatosplenomegaly and sudden death. In adults the iron deficiency anaemia may partly be due to malabsorption, for in some cases small bowel biopsy shows villous atrophy suggesting an association between coeliac disease and IPH.

499

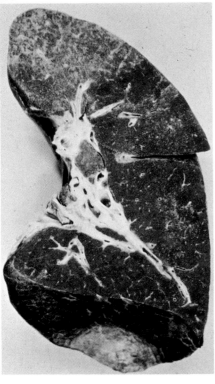

499 Idiopathic haemosiderosis. Whole lung section. The lungs and hilar glands are brick-red in colour from accumulation of haemosiderin.

500

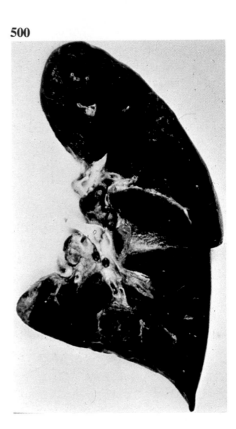

500 Idiopathic haemosiderosis. Whole lung section. The prussian blue reaction indicates the presence of haemosiderin.

501

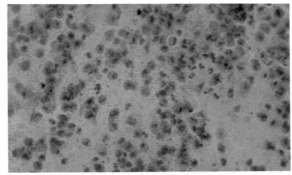

501 Haemosiderin-laden macrophages in sputum. These may be found in any condition causing intraalveolar pulmonary haemorrhage. The iron granules are stained green by Pearl's stain.

Amyloidosis

Diffuse amyloid deposition may involve the alveolar interstitium alone or as part of generalised amyloidosis. It is a rare condition.

502

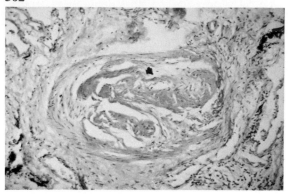

503

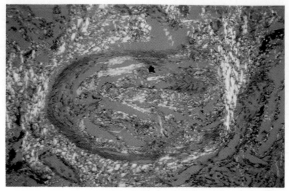

502 Nodular pulmonary amyloidosis with periarterial and alveolar capillary obliteration and alveolar thickening. *(H&E ×140)*

503 Birefringent amyloid fibres seen under polarised light. *(×40)*

Cryptogenic fibrosing alveolitis (CFA)

Synonyms: Alveolar interstitial fibrosis
Interstitial pneumonia
Hamman–Rich lung

The most common presenting symptoms are dyspnoea on exertion and a non-productive cough. Several causes of fibrosing alveolitis are increasingly well delineated and there remains a hard core of 'lone cryptogenic disease', in which two types seem to be emerging. One type is inflammatory, highly cellular and associated with circulating and fixed immune complexes, and with IgG deposition in the alveoli and capillaries. The other type is fibrotic, acellular and with no evidence of immune complex reactivity.

Serum antinuclear antibodies (ANA) are found in one-third of patients with CFA, and speckled and nucleolar ANA in six per cent.

Increased Clq binding levels are observed in 50 per cent of cases and even more frequently when there is also rheumatoid arthritis, the rheumatoid factor and IgG.

504

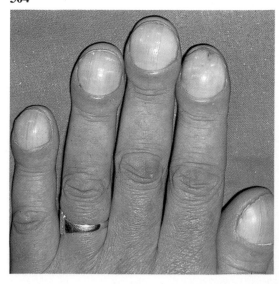

504 Severe clubbing of the fingers is characteristic (*see* table, page 230).

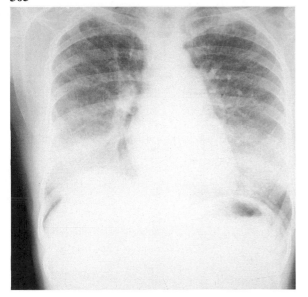

505 Bilateral lower zone pulmonary infiltration. The predominantly basal distribution differentiates CFA from sarcoidosis and extrinsic allergic alveolitis. Six months earlier inspiratory crackles were heard on auscultation of the lung bases and lung function showed a moderate restrictive defect.

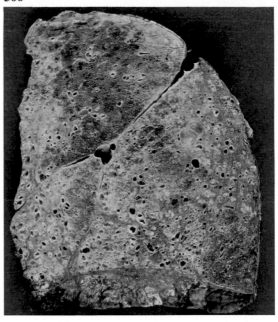

506 Honeycomb appearance of advanced cryptogenic fibrosing alveolitis. Necropsy specimen.

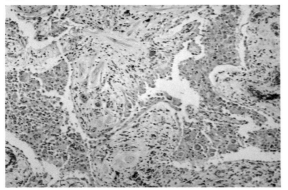

507 Desquamative interstitial pneumonia (DIP). Clumps of mononuclear cells fill the alveolar spaces. Lymphocytes and plasma cells are present in the interstitium which shows fibrosis with destruction of the lung architecture. *(H&E ×140)*

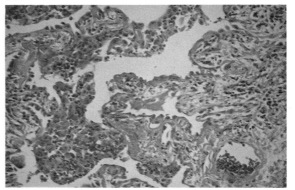

508 Interstitial pneumonia. Usual pattern. The alveolar walls are thickened by increased collagen and an inflammatory exudate of mononuclear cells. *(H&E ×100)*

The alveolar interstitium becomes disorganised as a result of a breakdown of collagen by a sustained enzymatic attack by collagenase. In the normal lung the ratio between Type I and II collagen is 2.5:1 but in cryptogenic fibrosing alveolitis the ratio rises to 5:1. Type I collagen is less yielding; this higher ratio is responsible for the loss of compliance and the restrictive defect. Instead of a regular arrangement of parallel crossbanded fibres of normal Type I collagen, the fibres are randomly twisted and frayed so that alveolar septa are patchily thickened or attenuated.

509

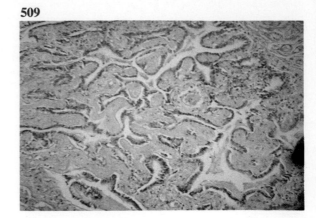

509 **End stage fibrosis** with loss of air space. The initial acute inflammatory features cannot be identified at this stage.

Pulmonary lymphangioleiomyomatosis

There is a proliferation of smooth muscle cells in lungs, lymphatics and lymph nodes in women of reproductive age, presenting with interstitial lung disease progressing to destructive cystic disease, emphysematous changes, spontaneous pneumothorax and chylous effusions.

The presenting symptoms are dyspnoea and haemoptysis.

510

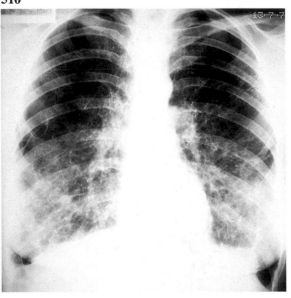

510 Progressive, fine reticulonodular infiltrates are characteristic but not specific. Most patients die from respiratory failure within 10 years of diagnosis.

511

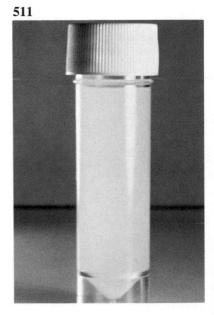

511 Chylous effusion is a diagnostic clue. Progesterone therapy is reported to improve the condition.

19 Sarcoidosis

Sarcoidosis is a multisystem disorder of unknown aetiology most commonly affecting adults, with a peak incidence in the third and fourth decades. The diagnosis is established by histological evidence of widespread non-caseating epithelioid cell granulomas in more than one organ and/or a positive Kveim-Siltzbach skin test. This skin test also reflects the activity of the disease. Immunological features are depression of delayed-type hypersensitivity, indicating T-cell anergy, and raised serum immunoglobulins, indicating B-cell overactivity (see Table on page 129). There may also be hypercalciuria with or without hypercalcaemia. The course and prognosis correlate with the mode of onset; an acute onset usually heralds a self-limiting course with spontaneous resolution, while an insidious onset may be followed by relentless progressive fibrosis (see Tables on pages 184 and 185).

Corticosteroids relieve symptoms and suppress inflammation and granuloma formation. Serum-angiotensin converting enzyme (SACE) is elevated in most patients and is a biochemical marker of activity. It falls towards normal with corticosteroid therapy and has proved a useful monitor of progress.

Although sarcoidosis is found worldwide, population studies reveal a variable prevalence. In England the prevalence overall is about 20 per 100,000; Irish women in London have a prevalence of 200 per 100,000. Sarcoidosis is more common in black patients in the USA, in the Caribbean and in Africa, where it may be confused with tuberculosis or leprosy.

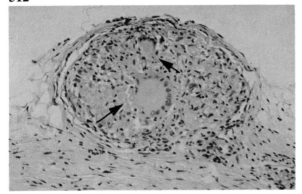

512 Sarcoid granuloma. The presence of granulomas is essential for the diagnosis of sarcoidosis. The distinguishing features are well-defined large epithelioid cells that stain pink with eosin, multinucleate giant cells (arrowed) and a surrounding rim of lymphocytes. Central necrosis is minimal. Granuloma formation may be induced by a wide variety of stimuli.

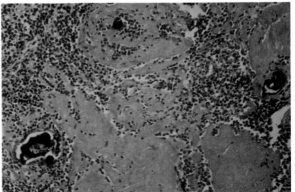

513 Inclusion bodies in granulomas. Three types are described:
1 Schaumann bodies. These are composed of calcium carbonate which impregnates the protein matrix. Their size is variable.
2 Residual bodies are doubly refractile and composed of calcium carbonate. They vary in size from 1 to $20\,\mu m$.
3 Asteroid bodies are 2 to $3\,\mu m$ in size.
None is unique to sarcoidosis. They are the debris of all metabolically active granulomas.

Table: Features of 818 patients with sarcoidosis.

Features	Number of patients	Percentage
Total	818	100
Women	500	61
Presentation under 40 years	604	74
Intrathoracic	700	88
Peripheral lymphadenopathy	225	27
Splenomegaly	101	12
Erythema nodosum	251	31
Other skin lesions	147	21
Ocular lesions	224	27
Nervous system	77	9
Parotid	52	6
Lacrimal	22	3
Bone	31	3
Heart	27	3
Kidney	10	1
Positive Kveim	550/657	84
Negative tuberculin	488/702	70
Hyperglobulinaemia	161/526	31
Hypercalcaemia	99/547	18
Corticosteroid therapy	344	42
Mortality caused by – Sarcoidosis – Other causes	25 23	3 3

Table: Acute v. chronic sarcoidosis.

Sarcoidosis	Acute (transient)	Chronic (persistent)
Age (years)	<30	>40
Onset	Abrupt	Insidious
Chest xray	Bilateral hilar lymphadenopathy	Pulmonary mottling
Eyes	Acute iritis, conjunctivitis, conjunctival nodules	Keratoconjunctivitis, chronic uveitis, glaucoma, cataract
Skin	Erythema nodosum, maculopapular rash, vesicular eruption	Lupus pernio, plaques, scars, keloids
Parotitis Lymphadenopathy Splenomegaly Bell's palsy	Usually transient	Rarely permanent
Bone cysts	No	Yes
Histology	Epithelioid and giant cells	Hyaline fibrosis
Lung biopsy	Positive	May be negative
Calcium metabolism	Hypercalcaemia, hypercalciuria	Nephrocalcinosis
Urinary hydroxyproline	Increased	Normal
Kveim–Siltzbach test	Positive	May be negative
Spontaneous remission	Frequent	Rare
Steroid therapy	Abortive effect	Symptomatic relief
Alternative drugs	Oxyphenbutazone	Chloroquine; potaba-methotrexate
Recurrence after steroid therapy	Rare	Frequent
Prognosis	Good	Poor

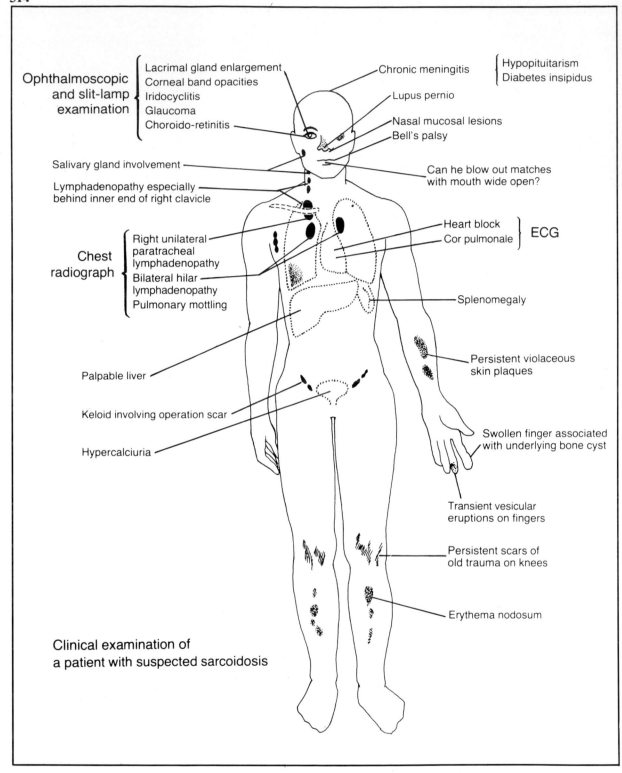

Ophthalmoscopic and slit-lamp examination
- Lacrimal gland enlargement
- Corneal band opacities
- Iridocyclitis
- Glaucoma
- Choroido-retinitis

Chronic meningitis

Hypopituitarism
Diabetes insipidus

Lupus pernio

Nasal mucosal lesions

Bell's palsy

Salivary gland involvement

Lymphadenopathy especially behind inner end of right clavicle

Can he blow out matches with mouth wide open?

Chest radiograph
- Right unilateral paratracheal lymphadenopathy
- Bilateral hilar lymphadenopathy
- Pulmonary mottling

Heart block
Cor pulmonale
ECG

Splenomegaly

Persistent violaceous skin plaques

Palpable liver

Keloid involving operation scar

Hypercalciuria

Swollen finger associated with underlying bone cyst

Transient vesicular eruptions on fingers

Persistent scars of old trauma on knees

Erythema nodosum

Clinical examination of a patient with suspected sarcoidosis

514   Clinical examination of patient with sarcoidosis.

Sarcoidosis – acute onset

The more abrupt the onset the better the prognosis.

515

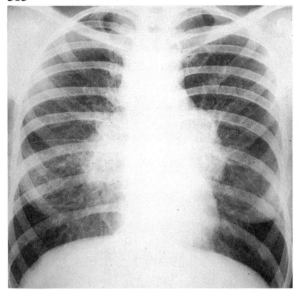

516

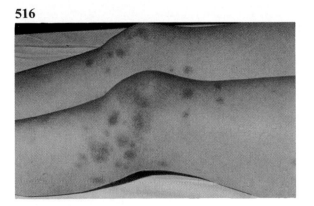

516 Erythema nodosum and arthralgia may be the symptoms of abrupt-onset sarcoidosis. Erythema nodosum is a non-specific hypersensitivity reaction provoked by many antigens (*see* page 95).

515 Bilateral hilar lymphadenopathy (BHL). The combination of erythema nodosum and hilar lymphadenopathy (Lofgren's syndrome) indicates acute exudative sarcoidosis. This acute-onset syndrome has a favourable outcome. Bilateral hilar lymphadenopathy is frequently a chance radiographic finding in a symptom-free patient. It may be expected to subside eventually in 60 per cent of patients.

517

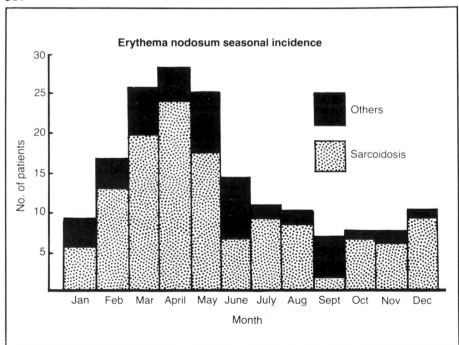

517 Erythema nodosum occurs most commonly in the spring season. It is most frequent in women of child-bearing age who are predominantly HLA-B8:A1.

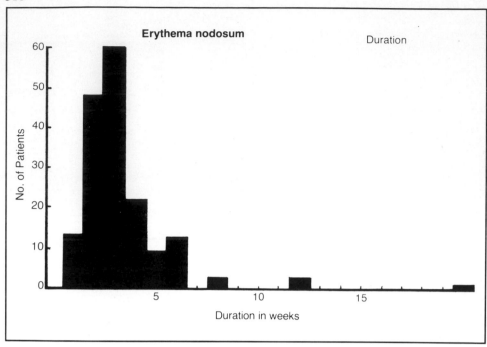

518 Erythema nodosum usually subsides within one month.

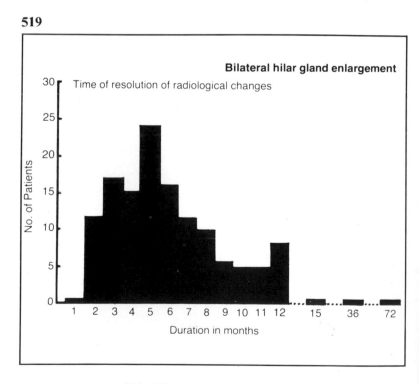

519 Hilar adenopathy usually resolves within one year.

520

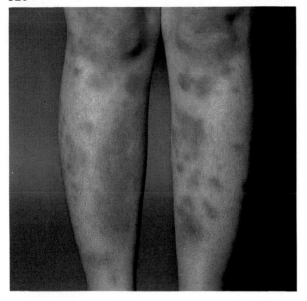

520 Erythema nodosum. As the condition subsides there is a play of colours from bright red to a brownish-yellowish discoloration resembling a bruise.

521

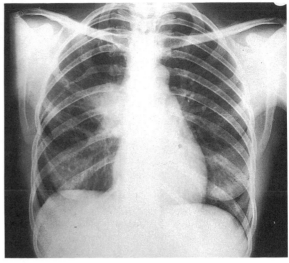

521 Hilar adenopathy may be unilateral when the differential diagnosis is tuberculosis or reticulosis. Histology of a lymph node is definitive. Unilateral hilar adenopathy caused by sarcoidosis is only one-tenth as frequent as its bilateral counterpart.

522

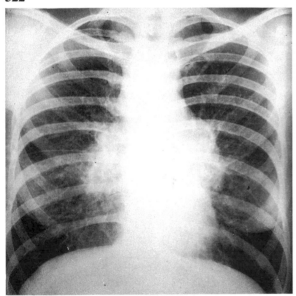

522 Hilar adenopathy and diffuse pulmonary infiltration – Stage II pulmonary sarcoidosis. Histological confirmation may be obtained by fibreoptic bronchoscopy or mediastinoscopy.

523

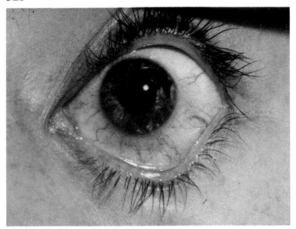

523 Iridocyclitis. Because sarcoidosis is a multisystem disorder, clinical examination must be thorough, including slit-lamp examination of the eyes.

524

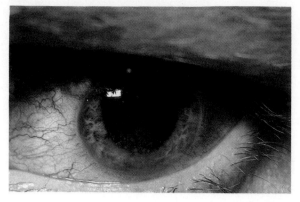

525

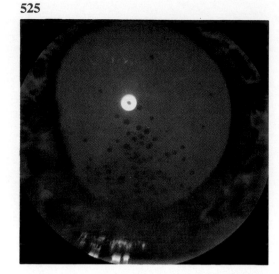

524 and 525 Keratic precipitates are best shown up by slit-lamp examination of the eyes.

526

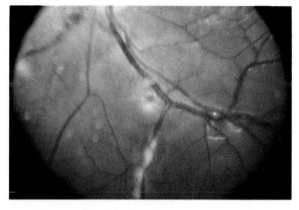

526 Acute choroidoretinitis with exudates and haemorrhages.

527

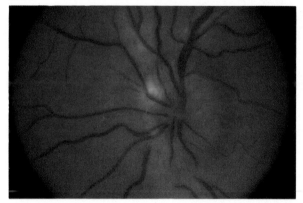

527 Papilloedema caused by sarcoidosis involving the optic nerve.

528

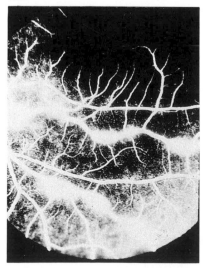

529

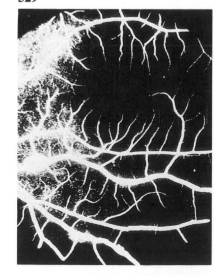

528 and 529 Vasculitis. Fluorescein angiography shows a fluffy appearance of the vessels which are the site of a vasculitis. Intravenous fluorescein leaks through diseased retinal vessels. There is considerable improvement after only three weeks of treatment with prednisolone (**529**).

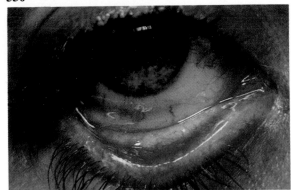

530 Conjunctival follicles in sarcoidosis. Biopsy revealed typical granulomas.

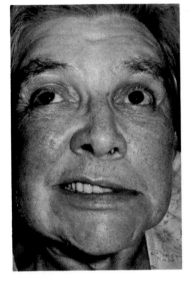

531 Left Bell's palsy. Lower motor neurone paralysis of the facial nerve, is usually unilateral and may be associated with uveitis and parotitis.

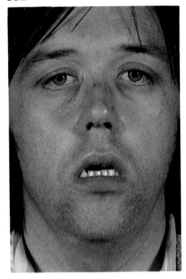

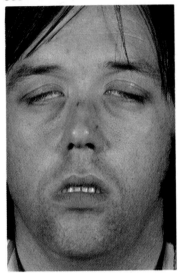

532 and 533 Bilateral facial nerve palsy resulting from sarcoidosis is rare. The patient is unable to close his lips or eyelids completely (533).

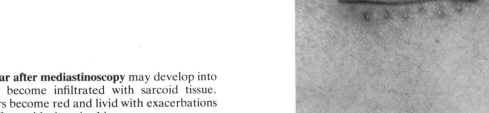

534 The scar after mediastinoscopy may develop into a keloid or become infiltrated with sarcoid tissue. Surgical scars become red and livid with exacerbations or activity of sarcoidosis as in this case.

Chronic sarcoidosis

The hallmarks of chronicity of sarcoidosis are chronic skin lesions and bone cysts. Their insidious onset suggests to the chest physician that the lung changes are also chronic, fibrotic and irreversible. The more insidious the onset the more protracted is the course of the disease.

535a and b Lupus pernio of the face is a most disfiguring form of chronic fibrotic sarcoidosis. It occurs predominantly in women in the fourth and fifth decades, presenting with nasal congestion or obstruction and followed by a purple macular eruption. It always involves nasal mucosa. This patient developed the condition in pre-cortisone days, so her bilateral uveitis progressed to blindness.

535a 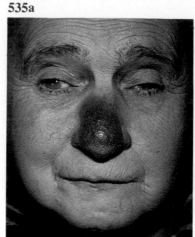 535b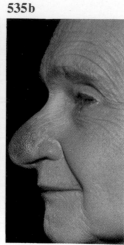

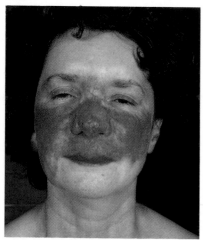

536 Extensive lupus pernio.

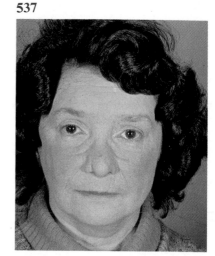

537 Cosmetic camouflage and corticosteroid drugs helped her appearance (same patient as **536**).

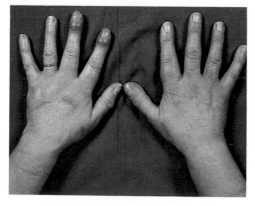

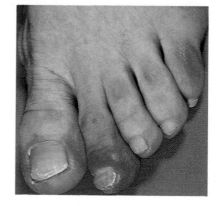

538 and 539 Lupus pernio of the extremities; smooth chilblain-like swellings are present on the fingers and one toe. The underlying phalange is usually involved and the nail often dystrophic. The same patient as in **536**.

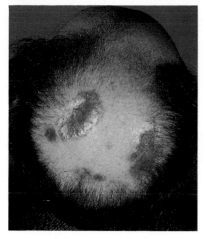

540 Plaques on the scalp. They were associated with progressive pulmonary fibrosis. A sarcoid skin plaque is generally rounded or oval, has a nodular slightly raised rim of a pinkish-brown encircling a clearer atrophic central area.

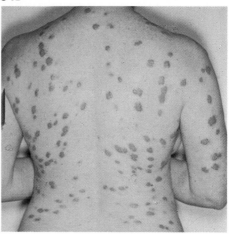

541 Small nodular infiltrations are commonly multiple affecting the arms and trunk. Skin plaques, like the accompanying lung lesions, persist indefinitely.

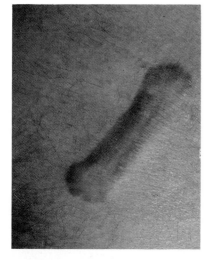

542 Stab wound infiltrated by sarcoid tissue.

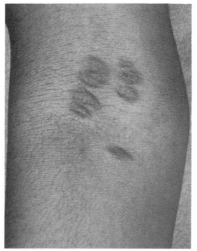

543 Sarcoid nodules at venesection sites in the antecubital fossa.

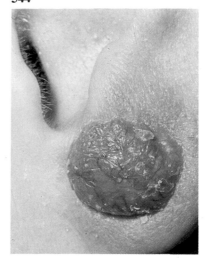

544 Sarcoid nodules at the site of earlobe piercing.

Infiltration of old scars may occur without other evidence of skin sarcoidosis. Its course follows that of the lung changes, the scar reverting to its normal flat pale state as the sarcoidosis activity wanes.

545

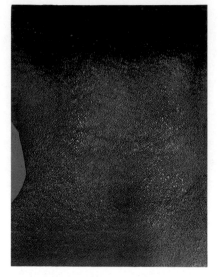

546

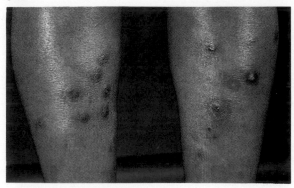

546 Nodular infiltrations of both legs. Little wonder that sarcoidosis has occasionally been subtitled 'European leprosy'.

545 Skin plaques caused by sarcoidosis on the nape of the neck often look like grains of salt.

547

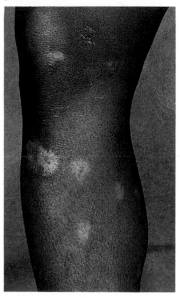

548

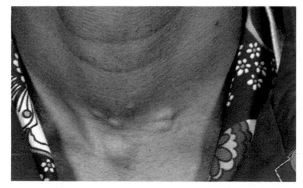

548 Subcutaneous nodules may be palpable in neck, trunk and limbs.

547 Nodular skin infiltration with sarcoidosis on leg. Healing has left depigmented areas, a complication which sometimes worries the patients more than the disease.

549

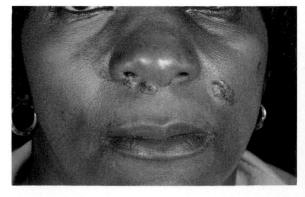

549 Skin plaques on face and right nostril. Plaques at the nostril are frequently associated with upper respiratory tract sarcoidosis.

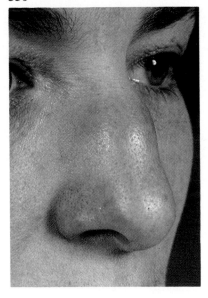

550 Sarcoidosis of upper respiratory tract is closely associated with lupus pernio. This patient with chronic sarcoidosis complained of nasal obstruction and a broadening of the bridge of her nose.

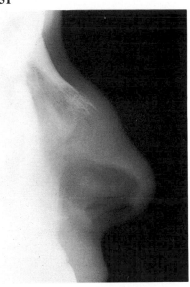

551 Sarcoidosis of the upper respiratory tract. The lateral radiograph shows osteoporotic changes in the nasal bones together with a soft-tissue swelling. The nasal symptoms responded to steroid therapy but there was no improvement in the disfiguring bone changes. (Same patient as **550**.)

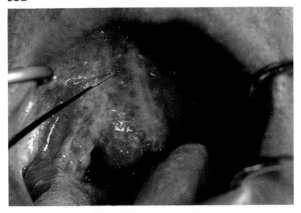

552 Extensive granulomatous lesions in the larynx and pharynx. The sarcoid granulomas have a cobblestone appearance. This patient presented with a sore throat and hoarseness.

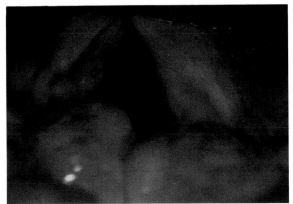

553 Sarcoid granulomas of larynx.

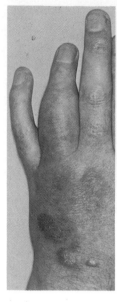

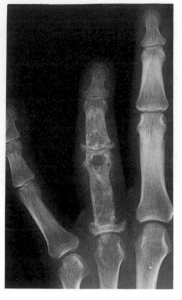

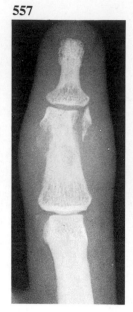

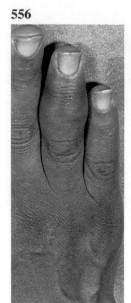

554 and 555 Chronic skin plaques and bone cysts. These bone changes rarely heal completely. There is residual shortening of the fourth digit, with a bone cyst involving the medulla of the proximal phalanx.

556 and 557 Phalangeal bone cysts causing 'sausage-shaped' swelling of one finger. Note the lytic lesion and fracture due to sarcoidosis.

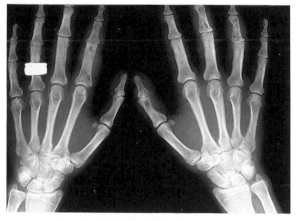

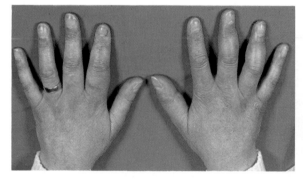

559 Phalangeal bone cysts. The fingers are swollen in this patient with chronic pulmonary sarcoidosis (same patient as **558**).

558 Phalangeal bone cysts. Lytic, reticular permeative and deforming lesions are shown on the xray.

560 Sarcoidosis of skeletal muscle. Contraction of the third, fourth and fifth fingers with a fixed flexion deformity at the wrist. Biopsy of the muscles of the forearm and biceps showed sarcoid granulomas. Symptomless infiltration of the muscles with sarcoid granulomas is sufficiently frequent for blind muscle biopsy to be worthwhile. Palpable muscle nodules and polymyositis are rare.

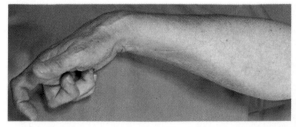

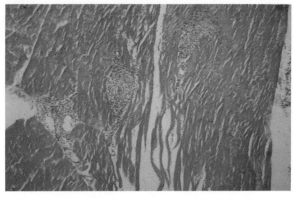

561 Sarcoid granuloma. Muscle biopsy.

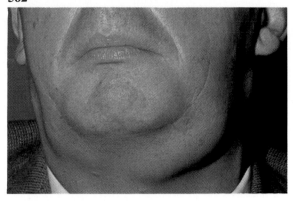

562 Submandibular lymphadenopathy. Enlargement of the superficial lymph nodes is a frequent finding during the course of sarcoidosis. The cervical lymph nodes are most commonly involved. Enlargement is seldom sufficient to attract the patient's attention. In this instance considerable enlargement of the submandibular glands is evident.

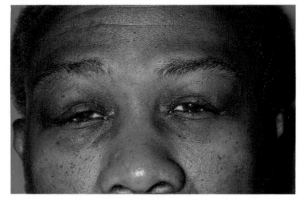

563 Lacrimal gland involvement is more frequent in black than in white persons. It may cause dry gritty eyes.

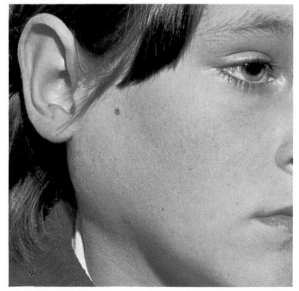

564 Parotid gland enlargement may be associated with anterior uveitis, fever, and facial nerve palsy (Heerfordt–Waldenström syndrome).

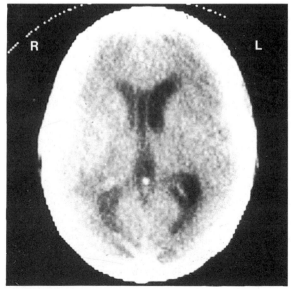

565 Internal hydrocephalus caused by ventricular blockage by gelatinous sarcoid tissue. An EMI-CAT scan revealed a dilated left ventricle in a patient who complained of severe unrelieved headaches.

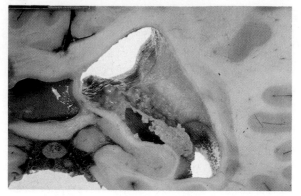

566

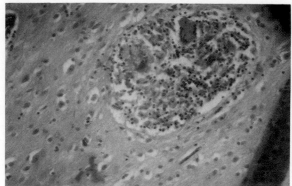

567

566 Cerebral sarcoidosis. Grape-like clusters of granulomas on the lateral ventricle, and also widely scattered elsewhere were revealed on necropsy. (Same patient as **565**.)

567 Cerebral sarcoidosis. Granulomas in brain tissue.

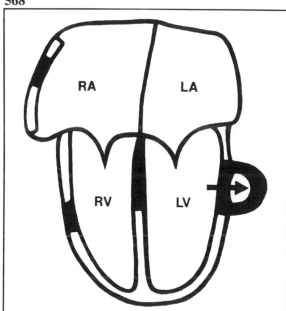

568

568 Involvement of the heart in sarcoidosis. The conduction bundle of His and the free ventricular wall of both ventricles are most frequently involved. Less commonly the right atrium may be affected. Cardiac involvement may be silent or become manifest as arrhythmias or myocardial infarction.

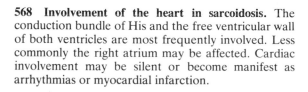

569

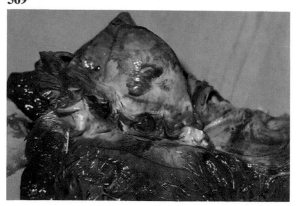

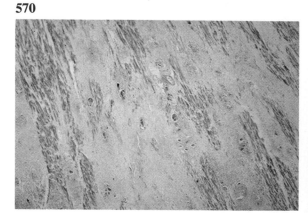

570

569 and 570 Myocardial sarcoidosis.

571

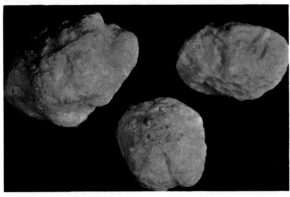

571 Renal calculi and nephrocalcinosis are complications of persistent hypercalciuria. The calcium stones caused acute renal colic. Hypercalciuria and hypercalcaemia reflect abnormal calcium metabolism which occurs in about 20 per cent of patients.

572

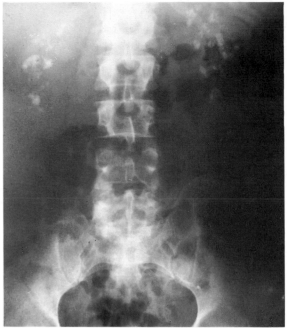

572 Nephrocalcinosis. A plain film of the abdomen.

Radiographic features

The three stages of intrathoracic involvement are shown in **573** to **575**.

573

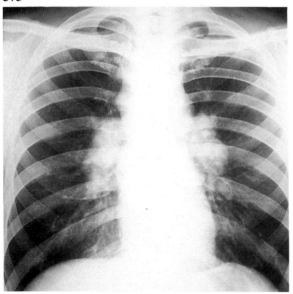

573 Bilateral hilar lymphadenopathy. Stage 1: This may be expected to subside in 60 per cent of patients.

574

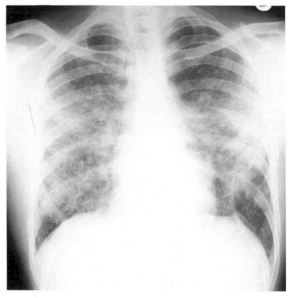

574 Bilateral hilar lymphadenopathy with pulmonary infiltration. Stage 2: This subsides in 40 per cent of patients.

575

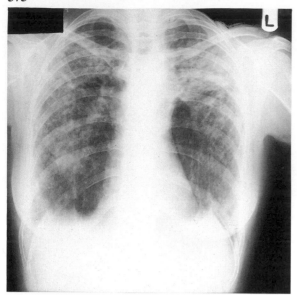

575 Diffuse pulmonary infiltration with or without pulmonary fibrosis and bullae formation. Stage 3: Subsequent resolution occurs in about 38 per cent of patients overall but no resolution can occur if the lungs are fibrotic.

576

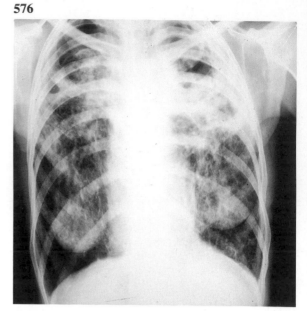

576 Extensive upper lobe fibrosis may give rise to bullae.

577

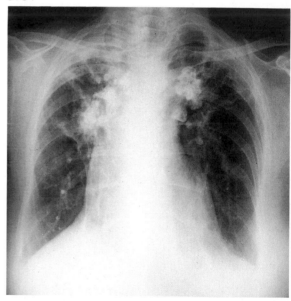

577 Pulmonary fibrosis and bulla formation.

578

578 Chronic fibrotic sarcoidosis with bilateral upper lobe shrinkage. The hilar glands have calcified. This patient also developed nephrocalcinosis and some renal impairment.

Diagnosis of sarcoidosis

The diagnosis of sarcoidosis is established most securely when clinicoradiographic patterns of disease are supported by histological evidence of widespread epithelioid-cell granulomas in more than one organ.

Biopsy material may be obtained from skin or lymph node if they are clinically involved or from the lung by fibreoptic bronchoscopy. Sarcoid granulomas may also be obtained by blind aspiration of the liver, muscle, lung, spleen, gum or salivary gland.

579

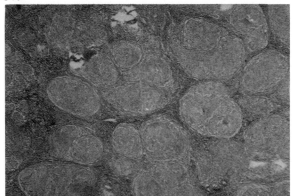

579 Scalene node biopsy specimen. Lymph node tissue may also be obtained by mediastinoscopy.

580

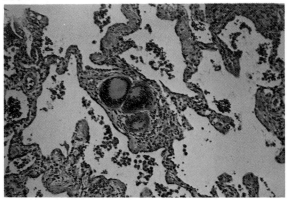

580 Bronchoscopic transbronchial lung biopsy is likely to show granulomas in 80 per cent of patients with active sarcoidosis.

581

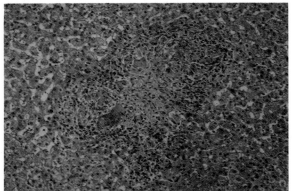

581 Liver granulomas found on serial sections of a specimen may be expected in 66 per cent of patients.

582

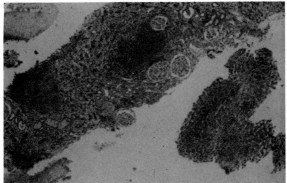

582 Kidney biopsy shows sarcoid tissue. Inadvertently the needle puncturing the kidney also punctured the liver and aspirated both kidney and liver. This specimen, showing sarcoid granulomas in both kidney and liver, is unique because it was achieved with one needle in a single biopsy. The fact that sarcoid granulomas are present in two different organs emphasises the multisystem nature of sarcoidosis.

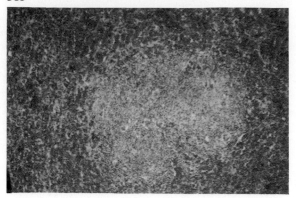

583 Sarcoid granuloma in pituitary gland. Diabetes insipidus is a rare complication of pulmonary sarcoidosis. The differential diagnosis is histiocytosis X (*see* page 178).

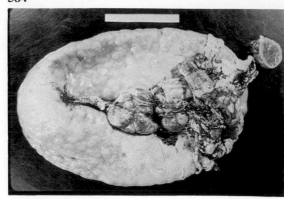

584 Human sarcoid spleen. The spleen is enlarged and infiltrated by sarcoid granulomas which have produced the surface's nodularity.

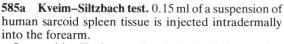

585a Kveim–Siltzbach test. 0.15 ml of a suspension of human sarcoid spleen tissue is injected intradermally into the forearm.

In a positive Kveim reaction the initial inflammation is slowly replaced by a raised red papule. Four to six weeks after injection a 3 mm to 4 mm Hayes–Martin drill biopsy is taken of the full thickness of the dermis at the test site.

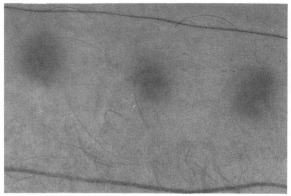

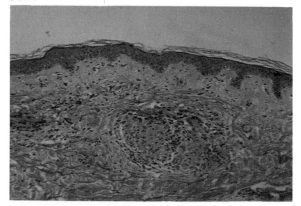

585b Positive Kveim–Siltzbach test. Sarcoid-like granulomas are seen when the core of tissue is subjected to serial section. A positive Kveim–Siltzbach skin test occurs in about three-quarters of patients.

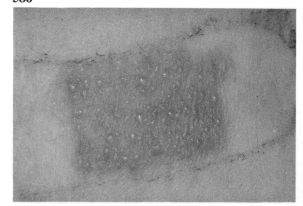

586 Dinitrochlorobenzene (DNCB) skin test. Cell-mediated immunity to all antigens is reduced in sarcoidosis, but is not so profound as occurs in malignant lymphomatous diseases. This vigorously positive DNCB skin test proclaims efficient T cells in a patient whose sarcoidosis has been cured.

Bronchial lavage

Cells and protein may be harvested from the lower respiratory tract by instilling sodium chloride 0.9 per cent solution through a fibreoptic bronchoscope or catheter and immediately suctioning the fluid back into a container.

Bronchial lavage recovers cells and proteins present on the epithelial surface of the lower respiratory tract which compare closely with the cellular and protein constituents obtained by open-lung biopsy.

In interstitial lung disease the differential count allows disorders to be broadly separated into those with high lymphocyte ratios and those with elevated neurophil ratios. High lymphocyte ratios are found in extrinsic allergic alveolitis or sarcoidosis and high neutrophil ratios in idiopathic pulmonary fibrosis and asbestosis.

587a **Bronchial lavage from normal lung.** The differential cell counts from lavage of a normal non-smoking adult reveals 93 per cent macrophages, 6 per cent lymphocytes, and only 1 per cent neutrophils. The average total cell count is from 5 to 10^6 cells per 100 ml of lavage. A larger number of cells is obtained from smokers' lungs containing 'activated macrophages' and an excess of neutrophils. (Arrow indicates macrophage.)

587b **Bronchial lavage from active Stage II sarcoidosis.** This differential count showed 55 per cent lymphocytes, 39 per cent macrophages and 6 per cent neutrophils. The unexpected finding of an elevated lymphocyte ratio suggests a granulomatous disorder.

In both sarcoidosis and extrinsic allergic alveolitis the lymphocytes found in the lungs are predominantly T lymphocytes. (Arrow indicates lymphocyte.)

587a

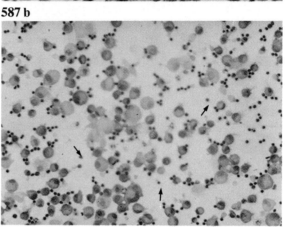

587b

Biochemical markers in sarcoidosis
Serum angiotensin-converting enzyme, transcobalamin II and lysozyme activity are all elevated in patients with active sarcoidosis. Measurement provides supporting but not specific diagnostic information.

588 Serum angiotensin-converting enzyme (SACE). Changes in SACE activity with steroid therapy are shown in a 32–year–old Afro-Caribbean woman with histologically proven pulmonary sarcoidosis. SACE monitors progress for it falls towards normal when steroid therapy suppresses activity of the granulomas. It also heralds relapses in the patient who is no longer having steroid therapy.

588

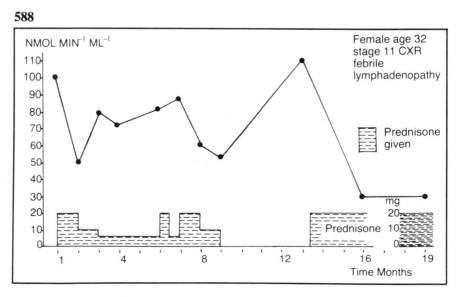

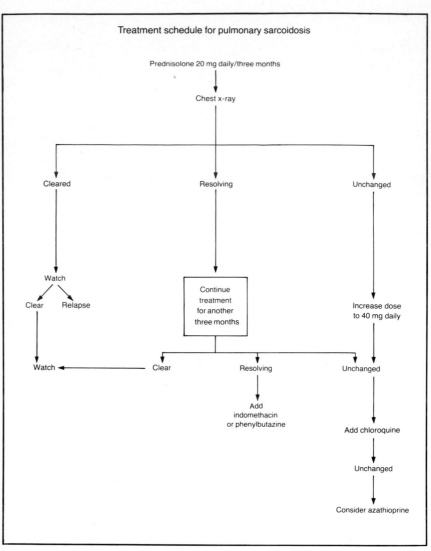

Treatment schedule for pulmonary sarcoidosis

Prednisolone 20 mg daily/three months

Chest x-ray

| Cleared | Resolving | Unchanged |

Cleared → Watch → Clear / Relapse → Watch

Resolving → Continue treatment for another three months

Unchanged → Increase dose to 40 mg daily

Continue treatment for another three months → Clear → Watch

Continue treatment for another three months → Resolving → Add indomethacin or phenylbutazine

Continue treatment for another three months → Unchanged

Increase dose to 40 mg daily → Unchanged → Add chloroquine → Unchanged → Consider azathioprine

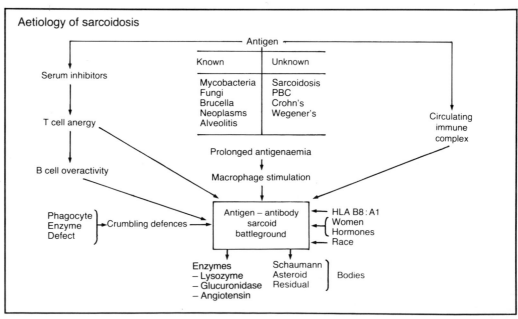

Aetiology of sarcoidosis

Antigen

Serum inhibitors

T cell anergy

B cell overactivity

Known	Unknown
Mycobacteria	Sarcoidosis
Fungi	PBC
Brucella	Crohn's
Neoplasms	Wegener's
Alveolitis	

Prolonged antigenaemia

Macrophage stimulation

Circulating immune complex

Phagocyte Enzyme Defect → Crumbling defences → Antigen – antibody sarcoid battleground ← HLA B8 : A1 / Women / Hormones / Race

Enzymes
– Lysozyme
– Glucuronidase
– Angiotensin

Schaumann
Asteroid
Residual } Bodies

Table: Differences between sarcoidosis and tuberculosis.

Features	Sarcoidosis	Tuberculosis
Age incidence (years)	20 to 50	Over 50
Fever	Rare	Common
Erythema nodosum	Common	Rare
Uveitis Skin involvement Enlarged parotids Bone cysts	Common	Very rare
Ulceration and sinuses	No	Common
Involvement of: Pleura Peritoneum Pericardium Meninges Small intestine	Very rare	Common
Caseation	Minimal	Maximal
Acid-fast bacilli	Absent	Present
Tuberculin test	Negative in 65 per cent	Positive in most
Kveim–Siltzbach test	Positive in most	Negative
Hypercalcaemia	Yes	No
Hypercalciuria	Yes	No
Angiotensin-converting enzyme	Positive	Negative
Calcification	No	Yes
Hilar lymphadenopathy	Bilateral	Unilateral
Pulmonary cavities	Rare, late	Common, early
Ghon focus	No	Yes
Corticosteroids	Helpful	Harmful alone
Antituberculous drugs	Unhelpful	Treatment of choice

20 Chronic bronchitis and emphysema

Chronic bronchitis is defined functionally as the occurrence of cough and phlegm on most days for at least three months in the year for two successive years.

The primary pathological abnormality is hypertrophy of the bronchial mucus glands and variable impairment of mucociliary clearance.

The symptoms should not be caused by bronchiectasis, tuberculosis or other specific cause. Changes in the bronchi may occur, leading to a sequence of permanent expiratory airflow limitation, hyperinflation of the lungs and finally impairment of gas exchange.

Emphysema is defined anatomically and is said to be present where there is enlargement of air spaces beyond the terminal non-respiratory bronchioles, usually with destruction of lung tissue. The diagnosis covers a number of abnormalities which can only be identified with certainty by histological examination.

Severe airflow obstruction with breathlessness is a feature of both conditions.

The definitions are not exclusive, for patients with chronic obstructive bronchitis may respond in part to treatment with bronchodilating drugs, while most patients with emphysema develop chronic bronchitis with cough and sputum.

Numerous studies have related the presence of adult respiratory symptoms to cigarette smoking, atmosphere pollution, certain dusty occupations, recurrent childhood respiratory tract infections and genetic factors.

Chronic bronchitis

These patients, who may not be very breathless, tend to be obese, centrally cyanosed and show signs of 'cor pulmonale'. In severe disease the arterial PO_2 is low leading to compensatory polycythaemia. Chronic elevation of the arterial PCO_2 leads to a compensatory respiratory acidosis.

589

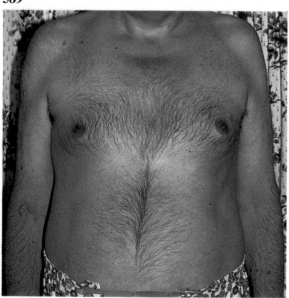

589 Chronic bronchitis. Cyanosed obese patient receiving treatment for central congestive cardiac failure. 'Blue and bloated' aptly describes these patients' appearance.

590

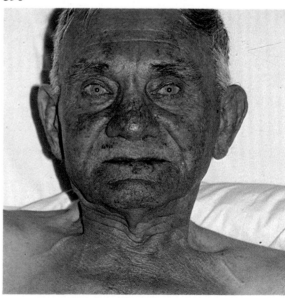

590 Chronic bronchitis. Central cyanosis and engorged neck veins caused by secondary right heart failure – cor pulmonale.

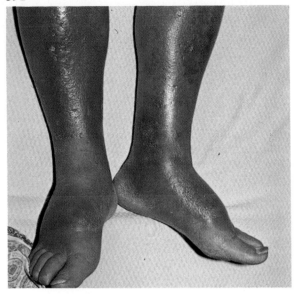

591 Chronic bronchitis. Cor pulmonale with gross peripheral oedema.

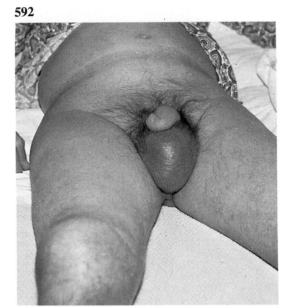

592 Chronic bronchitis. Ascites with scrotal and genital oedema. Breathlessness was not severe in spite of severe hypoxia and elevation of the arterial carbon-dioxide tension.

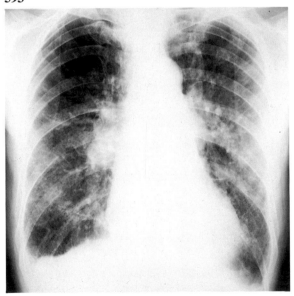

593 Chronic bronchitis. Cor pulmonale. The radiographic features are of cardiomegaly, dilatation of the proximal pulmonary vessels and bilateral pleural effusions. The same patient as in **591** and **592**.

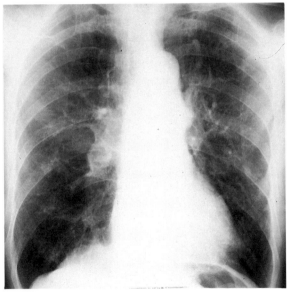

594 Chronic bronchitis. Cor pulmonale. Treatment for cor pulmonale with diuretics produced considerable improvement. The pleural effusions have cleared and the dilated heart is smaller.

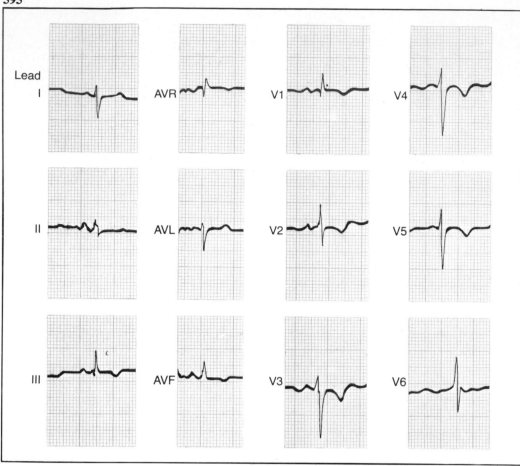

595

Lead I   AVR   V1   V4

II   AVL   V2   V5

III   AVF   V3   V6

595 Electrocardiogram of patient (593 and 594). The criteria for right ventricular hypertrophy are an R wave of 7 mm or more in V_1, a combined voltage of R wave in V_1 and S wave in V_6 of 10 mm or more, an R wave taller than the S wave in V_6 and right axis deviation. P. pulmonale is a frequent finding.

596 Pursed lip expiration is a common feature in severe airflow obstruction. In an attempt to prevent premature airways collapse and air trapping the patient maintains an elevated intrathoracic pressure by exhaling slowly against a raised intralaryngeal or oral pressure. The lips are cyanosed.

597 Peripheral signs of carbon dioxide retention include dilated veins, a bounding pulse and flapping tremor of the dorsiflexed outstretched hands similar to that seen in hepatic encephalopathy. Peripheral cyanosis always accompanies central cyanosis and may be seen in the nail vascular beds.

596

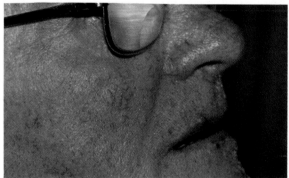

597

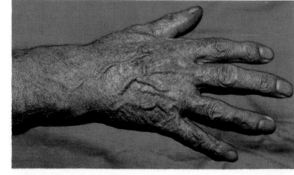

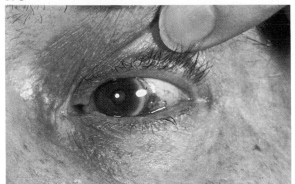

598 Subconjunctival flame-shaped haemorrhage indicates transient elevation of the venous pressure during a bout of coughing. Cough syncope in which the patient faints during a bout of coughing also indicates raised venous and intrathoracic pressure with transient reduction in cardiac output, cerebral hypoxia and transient loss of consciousness.

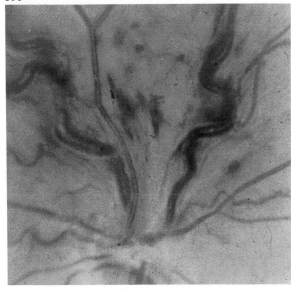

599 Fundal vessels dilate with elevation of the arterial carbon dioxide tension (PCO_2) but papilloedema is uncommon. The cerebral vessels dilate in response to PCO_2 elevation and the patient may complain of headache.

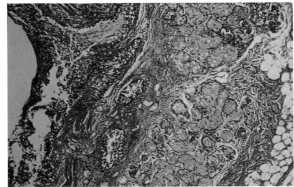

600 Mucous gland hyperplasia and chronic inflammation. The ratio of the glandular layer to the total bronchial wall thickness may increase by 30 to 40 per cent. Haemophilus influenzae and Streptococcus pneumoniae are the common infective organisms found in the mucopurulent sputum of the bronchitic. *(Alcian blue ×100)*

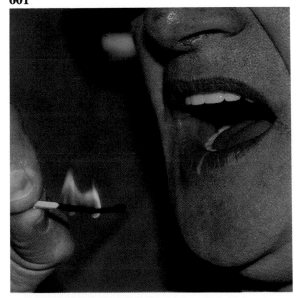

601 Bedside lung function tested with a lighted match. Airflow obstruction prevents the patient exhaling rapidly enough through the open mouth to extinguish the flame.

209

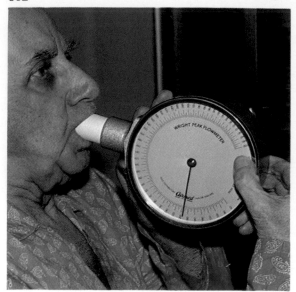

602 Measurement of peak expiratory flow. This is a convenient test for routine assessment.

Emphysema

Patients suffering from emphysema tend to be thin, breathless at rest and are aptly described as 'pink puffers'. Arterial desaturation may occur on effort but in contrast to patients with chronic bronchitis a normal sensitivity to carbon dioxide remains.

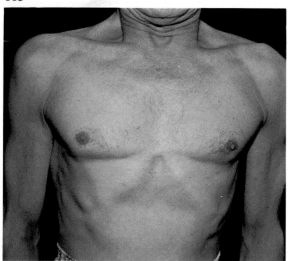

603 **Barrel-shaped chest in emphysema** is a sign of hyperinflation and air trapping. The absence of cyanosis, horizontal ribs, prominent sternal angle and increased anteroposterior diameter of the chest are characteristic.

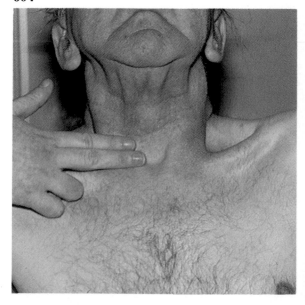

604 **Tracheal tug.** Inspiratory shortening of the distance between the thyroid cartilage and the suprasternal notch is attributed to contraction of a low flat diaphragm. The distance between the circothyroid cartilage and the suprasternal notch measures the length of the trachea outside the thorax and is normally at least three finger widths in vertical distance.

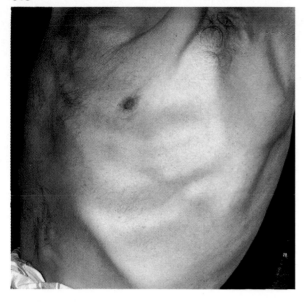

605 Indrawing of the intercostal spaces is another sign of hyperinflation of the chest.

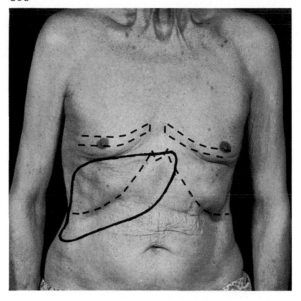

606 Emphysema. The liver is displaced downwards so that the lower edge is palpable. The upper border of the liver is normally at the level of the fifth rib.

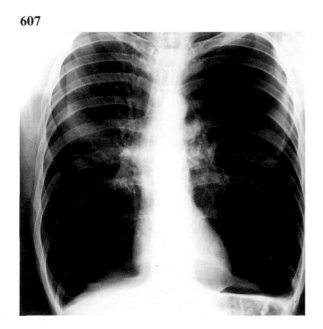

607 Emphysema. The PA xray shows hyperinflation with low flat diaphragms at the level of the eleventh rib and oligaemia caused by loss of the pulmonary vessels.

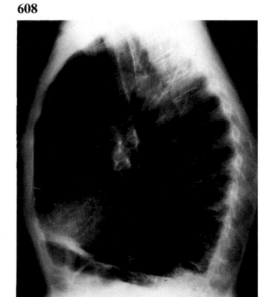

608 The lateral xray shows an increased retrosternal air space and a very deep posteroanterior diameter. The heart is of normal size.

609

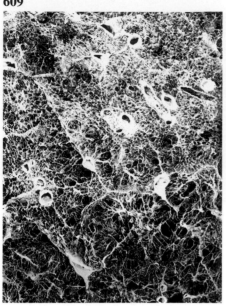

609 Pan-lobular emphysema (panacinar). The air spaces beyond the terminal bronchioles are destroyed in a relatively uniform manner throughout the affected lobule. Contrast the extensively destroyed alveolar walls in the lower portion of the photograph with the more normal appearance above. *(Barium sulphate impregnation ×15).*

610

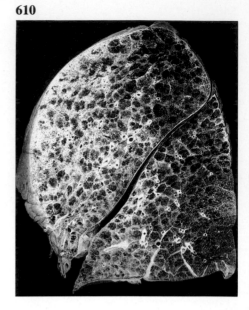

610 Centrilobular emphysema (centracinar). This form of emphysema involves air spaces in the centre of lobules. This whole left lung section shows patchy centrilobular emphysema.

Alpha₁ antitrypsin deficiency

This inherited metabolic deficit is associated with basal pulmonary emphysema in adults and neonatal hepatitis and cirrhosis in children. Alpha₁ antitrypsin is an antiproteolytic factor which neutralises collagen, destroying proteolytic substances secreted from inflammatory cells in the alveoli.

611

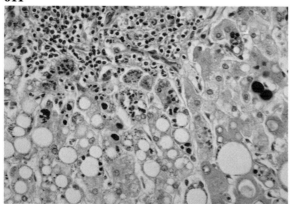

611 Alpha₁ antitrypsin deficiency. A liver biopsy from a cirrhotic patient shows brightly staining diastase resistant inclusions concentrated around the portal tracts. Release into the circulation is defective and the red granular inclusions represent accumulated alpha₁ antitrypsin in the liver.

612

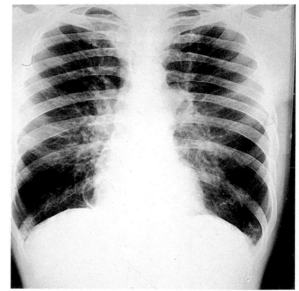

612 Alpha₁ antitrypsin deficiency. Severe predominantly basal emphysema in a 37 year old man. Death in 'cor pulmonale' occurred soon after. Homozygous patients have little if any circulating alpha₁ antitrypsin and run a high risk of developing emphysema.

Results from spirometric tests

The simple measurement of forced expiratory volume in one second (FEV_1) and forced vital capacity (FVC) gives valuable information. A forced delivery of air from maximum inspiration to maximum expiration (FVC) is mandatory and therefore patient co-operation is essential.

The results of spirometry can be compared with tabulated predicted values dependent upon age, sex and height.

Three broad categories of result may be obtained.

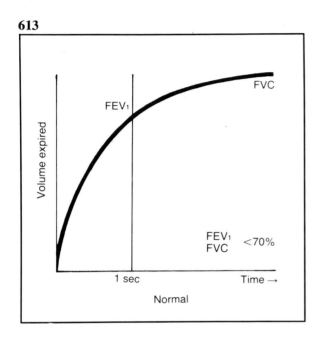

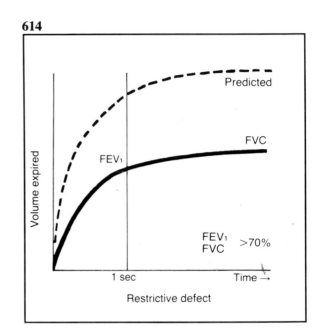

613   Normal spirogram. Values of FEV_1 and FVC at predicted level and FEV_1/FVC ratio 70 per cent.

614   Restrictive defect. Reduction of FEV_1 and FVC but preservation of a normal FEV_1/FVC ratio. Restrictive lung diseases may be divided into two groups – (i) extrapulmonary restriction caused by chest-wall rigidity, respiratory muscle weakness or pleural thickening (ii) intrapulmonary restriction caused by lung fibrosis.

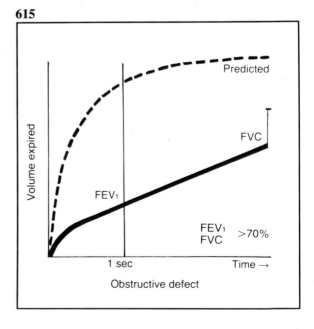

615   Obstructive defect. The FEV_1 and FEV_1/FVC ratio are considerably reduced. The forced expiratory time required to reach FVC is prolonged. This picture is seen in chronic airflow limitation and bronchospasm.

21 Pulmonary embolism and infarction

Pulmonary embolism is the impaction of thrombus or foreign matter in the pulmonary vascular bed. Pulmonary infarction is the pathological change which develops in the lung as a result of a pulmonary embolus. Thrombo-embolism usually follows deep-vein thrombosis of the thigh and leg veins or the pelvic veins. Less commonly, thrombi may embolise from axillary and arm veins or the right heart cavities. The three factors thought to predispose to vascular thrombosis are reduction in blood flow, damage to vessel walls and increased coagulability of blood. The contributing factors include bed rest and immobility; surgery, trauma and burns; previous venous thrombosis and cardiac disease; obesity and paralytic disorders. The single most important diagnostic factor is the awareness of the possibility of embolism in these high-risk groups (*see* Table) for the various tests tend to be nonspecific (*see* Table). Uncommon non-thrombotic embolism may be caused by air, fat, malignant cells, amniotic fluid, parasites and foreign material.

Table: Clinical features of pulmonary thromboembolism.

Type	Symptoms and signs	Remarks
Silent	Asymptomatic	Probably more frequent than we realise
Without infarction	Breathlessness Tachycardia Anxiety Restlessness	Usually transient
With infarction	Dyspnoea Pleural pain Haemoptysis Friction rub Fever Bronchospasm	If you wait for these features you will miss perhaps 60 per cent of patients with embolism
With haemodynamic impairment	Angina Tachycardia P2 + + Gallop rhythm JVP Hypotension Cyanosis Syncope	This means obstruction of 30 to 50 per cent of pulmonary vascular bed

Table: Value of tests for thromboembolism.

Test	Abnormal features	Remarks
Chest xray	Elevated diaphragm Wedge-shaped opacity Atelectasis Dilated azygos vein Serosanguineous pleural effusions	It may be normal after acute embolism
Electrocardiogram	Sinus tachycardia S1, Q3, T3, P. pulmonale Right axis deviation Incomplete RBBB T wave inversion Arrhythmias	Chest xray and electrocardiogram should be routine
Radioactive scanning	Abnormal lung perfusion 'Hot' and 'cold' spots	Unfortunately non-specific and too many false-positives. Don't do it if chest xray abnormal. A normal perfusion scan with a normal chest xray rules out pulmonary embolism.
Pulmonary arteriogram	Intravascular filling defect or vessel 'cut-off'	Reliable but unfortunately an invasive technique
Leucocyte count	Under 15,000	If over 15,000 consider bacterial sepsis
Isoenzyme pattern	Normal	Only helpful in distinguishing embolism from myocardial infarction
Arterial oxygen tension	Decreased	Non-specific
Alveolar-arterial oxygen tension difference	Increased difference	Even more sensitive but still non-specific

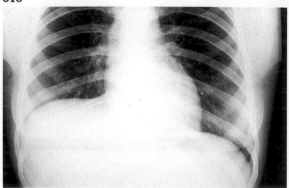

616 Pulmonary embolism in a 23-year-old woman using the contraceptive pill. The abrupt onset of right-sided pleuritic chest pain and severe dyspnoea led to an xray showing elevation of the right diaphragm. Three recent episodes of breathlessness and hyperventilation had incorrectly been attributed to anxiety.

617

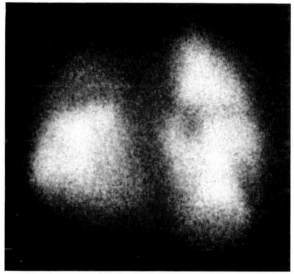

617 Technetium 99m (TC 99m) labelled albumen microsphere perfusion scan. A wedge-shaped perfusion defect is evident in the right lower lobe and there are extensive perfusion defects in the radiographically normal left upper and lower lobes.

618

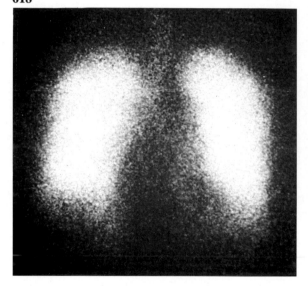

618 Krypton 81 ventilation scan. The radioactive emission is evenly distributed throughout both lung fields. The perfusion scan defects do not match with the ventilation scan and are typical of multiple pulmonary embolism.

619

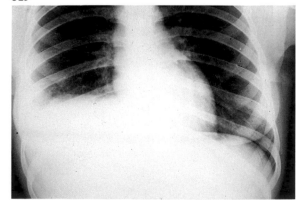

619 Pleural effusion formed by the sixth day. Pulmonary infarction is common when minor pulmonary arteries are occluded. Such an event is not associated with a significant circulatory disturbance.

620

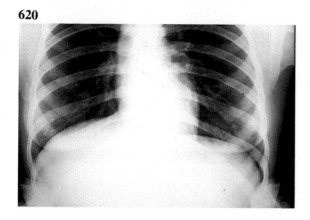

621

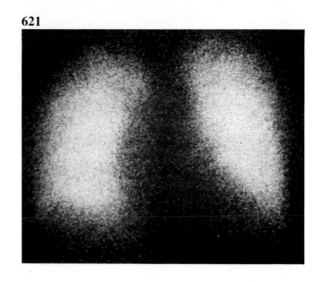

620 and 621 The xray and isotope perfusion scan (**Technetium 99m**) were normal after six weeks' therapy with anticoagulants.

622

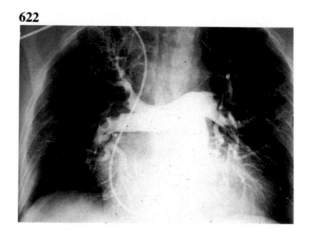

622 Acute massive pulmonary embolism. The pulmonary angiogram shows good filling of the right upper and left lower lobe vessels only. The remaining vessels show varying degrees of embolic occlusion. A repeat angiogram two months later showed normal perfusion.

623

623 Acute massive pulmonary embolism. Chest xray. The heart is large and the lung fields oligaemic (same patient as **622**.)

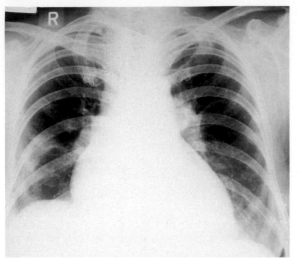

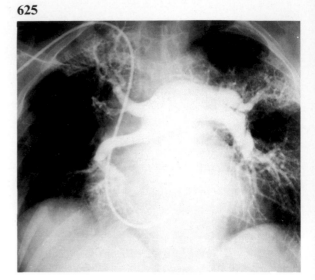

624 Chronic pulmonary embolism. Prominent pulmonary arteries and the huge cardiac silhouette are caused by pulmonary hypertension. This 45-year-old man was a chronic respiratory invalid after three major and repeated minor pulmonary emboli. Right heart catheter studies showed a right ventricular pressure 88/6 and pulmonary artery pressure of 88/30.

625 Chronic pulmonary embolism. Pulmonary angiogram. Perfusion to the right middle and lower lobes and left upper lobes is obstructed. The left proximal pulmonary artery is dilated secondary to pulmonary hypertension. (Same patient as **624**.)

626 The electrocardiogram of (622) shows tachycardia, a right axis shift, the appearance of an S wave in lead I and a Q wave with T wave inversion in lead III. T wave inversion and partial right bundle branch block are seen in $V_1–V_4$.

626

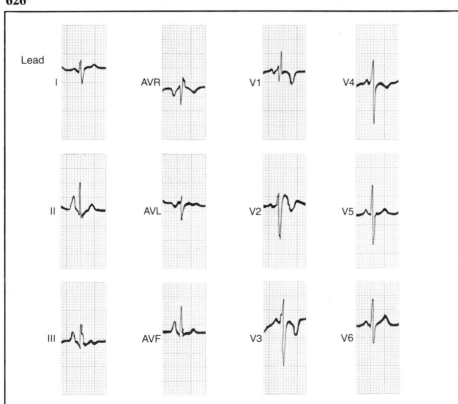

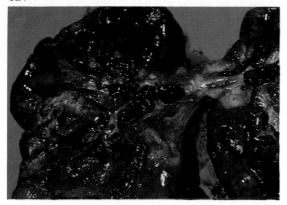

627 **Embolism in the main pulmonary artery** and its major branches occluded the circulation eight days after hysterectomy. Necropsy shows a granular laminated ante-mortem clot which had arisen from the pelvic veins. A smooth shiny post-mortem clot is present. The coiled thrombi, extracted at necropsy from the pulmonary artery corresponded in calibre to the leg veins from which they arose.

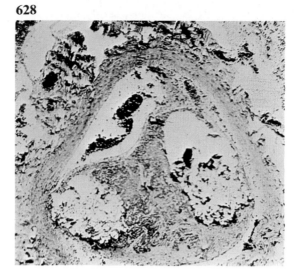

628 **Cotton fibre emboli** lying in a small pulmonary artery. A granulomatous foreign body reaction is stimulated and results in damage to the vessel wall and the ultimate extension of the lesion into the perivascular tissues. Schistosome eggs are similarly extruded through pulmonary vessel walls.

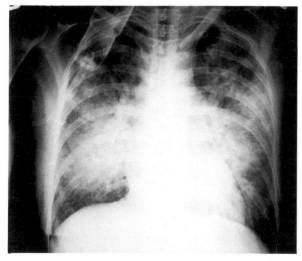

629 **Fat emboli in the lungs** can follow a fracture of the long bones. This woman fractured the neck of her femur in a road traffic accident. Forty-eight hours later, she was confused, cyanosed and had developed a petechial skin rash. The xray shows a pattern simulating pulmonary oedema. Fat droplets were present in the sputum and urine. This condition may also result from a jockey's riding injury.

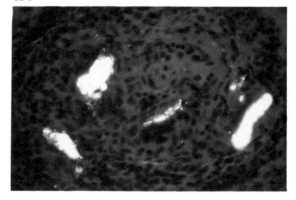

630 **Emboli in drug addict's lungs.** Lung biopsy showing a foreign body granuloma and birefringent particles under polarising light. The patient has diffuse interstitial lung disease. The high price and scarcity of illicit drugs lead to their adulteration with inert 'fillers' of starch, lactulose or talc. (*Polarised light H&E ×140*)

22 Respiratory failure

Respiratory failure may be said to be present if the lungs are unable to provide adequate aeration of the blood at a particular level of activity.

The limits defining this failure are an arterial oxygen tension (PaO_2) of less than 60 mm Hg (8kPa) and an arterial carbon dioxide tension ($PaCO_2$) of more than 50 mm Hg (6.7 kPa), the patient being at rest and breathing air at sea level.

O_2 dissociation curve

O_2 forms an easily reversible combination with haemoglobin (Hb). The saturation of arterial blood with a PaO_2 of 100 mm Hg is about 97.5 per cent while that of mixed venous blood with a PaO_2 of 40 mm Hg is about 75 per cent. Cyanosis is clinically apparent with a saturation of less than 85 per cent.

The curved shape of the O_2 dissociation curve is advantageous (*see* **631**). The flap top end tends to stabilise the quantity of oxygen in the arterial blood, while the steep middle part of the curve ensures that a large proportion of the oxygen which is carried by the blood is delivered to the tissues at a relatively high tension. The position of the O_2 dissociation curve is influenced by pH, PCO_2 and temperature; acidosis and fever increase the oxygen uptake in the tissues.

Respiratory failure may result from chemoreceptor or medullary respiratory centre depression, mechanical disorders limiting ribcage movement, physiological shunting with mismatch of ventilation and perfusion or anatomical shunting of blood through congenital cardiac defects. Failure, both acute and chronic, can be divided into two main groups according to the arterial PCO_2 level.

Type I **Hypoxaemia without hypercapnia**
Cardiogenic pulmonary oedema
Adult respiratory distress syndrome
Acute pneumonia
Pulmonary thromboembolism
Severe bronchial asthma
R-L shunts in congenital cardiac disease
R-L shunts in pulmonary arteriovenous malformation

Type II **Hypoxaemia with hypercapnia**
Primary alveolar hypoventilation
Chronic airflow obstruction
Respiratory sedative drugs
Ribcage trauma
Cerebrovascular disease – stroke, space occupying lesion
High spinal cord lesion or polyneuritis
Myopathies

631

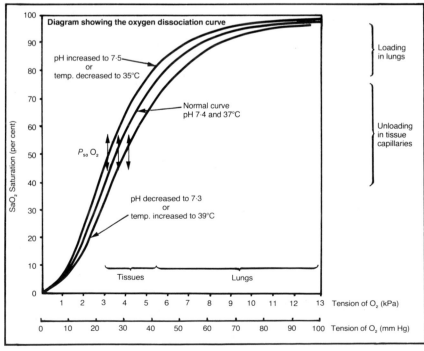

Adult respiratory distress syndrome

The adult respiratory distress syndrome (ARDS) is an important form of acute respiratory failure. There are many causes.

The syndrome is best recognised in patients who have suffered an acute often multisystem illness. Characteristically there is a short latent period of 12 to 24 hours between the primary event and the onset of dyspnoea, tachypnoea, a low arterial oxygen tension (PaO_2 <50 mm Hg) in spite of high inspired oxygen concentrations (FiO_2 >60 per cent) and diffuse patchy shadows on chest xray. The lung bases are often clear.

In defining ARDS it is important to exclude primary left ventricular failure and most forms of chronic lung disease.

Regardless of the mechanism of lung injury, non-cardiogenic pulmonary oedema develops secondary to an increase in the permeability of the alveolar capillary endothelium. Pneumocytes are damaged and surfactant synthesis reduced. The total respiratory compliance falls and inspiratory pressures required to inflate the stiff lungs are high. There are many similarities between ARDS and hyaline membrane disease of the newborn.

632 a

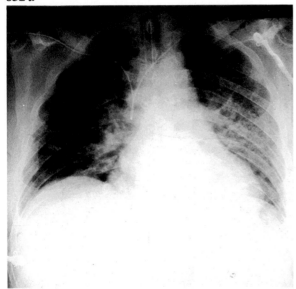

632a Adult respiratory distress syndrome – 1st day. Acute cyanosis and dyspnoea 12 hours after aspiration of gastric contents during grand mal epileptic convulsion. Before ventilation the arterial PO_2 was 3.9 kPa. An endobronchial tube, misplaced subclavian line and dense left lung alveolar infiltrate are present.

632b

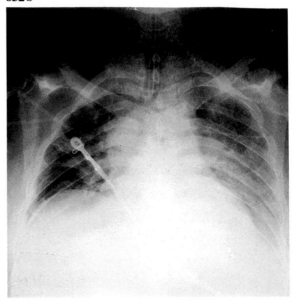

632b Adult respiratory distress syndrome – 5th day. Same patient as **631**. More extensive and bilateral alveolar infiltrate. Inspired O_2 tension of 60 per cent (FiO_2) was necessary to maintain an arterial PO_2 of 9 kPa. Death finally resulted from infection.

Table: Major factors associated with adult respiratory distress syndrome.

Pneumonia	Trauma
– viral	– fat emboli
– bacterial	– lung contusion
– fungal	– head and non-thoracic
– Pneumocystis carinii	injury
Gram-negative septicaemia	Liquid aspiration
	– gastric contents
Disseminated intravascular	– drowning
coagulation	
	Drug overdose

23 Tumours of the lung

Primary tumours

A wide range of tumours may arise in the lung, about 95 per cent of which are bronchial carcinomas. In economically developed countries the mortality rate from bronchial carcinoma has risen considerably during the past 40 years, accounting for one in 11 of all deaths in British males and 40 per cent of total male cancer deaths. The ratio of male to female lung cancer deaths has narrowed. More women die nowadays from oat-cell and squamous-cell carcinoma.

About 90 per cent of lung cancers are associated with cigarette smoking. The prevalence of small-cell and squamous-cell carcinomas is related to tobacco smoking, atmospheric pollution and some industrial processes. Adenocarcinoma may arise in lung scars caused by exposure to asbestos or healed tuberculosis. It is relatively more common in non-smokers and women. The survival statistics are gloomy for of any 100 newly diagnosed lung cancers, fewer than 10 patients will live five years. Eighty cases will be too advanced for surgical resection and most of these will be dead within three years. Twenty patients will have an operation of which six will be alive after five years (*see* table).

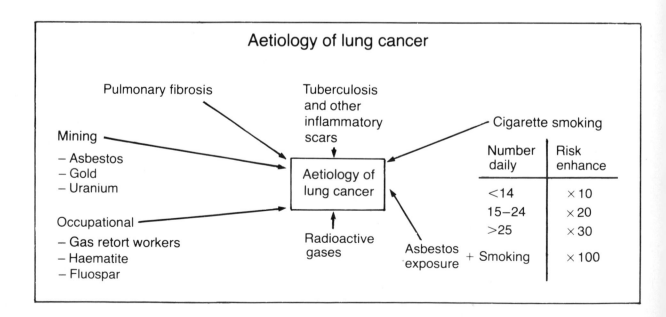

Table: Bronchial neoplasm. Clinical and hormonal manifestations.

Cell type (percentage frequency)	Clinical features	Hormone	Clinical and biochemistry	Metabolic therapy
Squamous 50 per cent	Slow growing. Finger clubbing and hypertrophic osteoarthropathy Hypercalcaemia	Parathormone	Often acute onset anorexia, nausea, vomiting, constipation, polyuria, polydipsia High plasma calcium, low normal phosphate, normal alkaline phosphatase Raised PTH and CEA Steroid suppression test (calcium falls)	Correct dehydration Calcitonin Mithramycin Prednisolone Prostaglandin inhibitors (aspirin and indomethacin)
Small (oat) 20 per cent	Rapid growing. Think of it in patients under 40 years of age. Occurs in large bronchi. Early lymphatic and haematogenous spread	ACTH increased in 29 per cent Cortisol increased in 50 per cent in 24 hours	Usually classical Cushing's syndrome absent Weakness myopathy Hypokalaemic alkalosis Loss of cortisol circadian variation Usually no suppression of plasma or urinary steroids with high-dose dexamethasone Metyrapone test usually shows autonomous secretion	Metyrapone ± replacement therapy with prednisolone Surgery/radiotherapy/ chemotherapy
		ADH inappropriate in 33 per cent	Drowsiness, confusion, fits Dilutional hyponatraemia Inappropriately high urine osmolality Water-load test – inability to excrete water	Water restriction Hypertonic saline (emergency) Demethylchlortetracycline Lithium
		Calcitonin increased in 65 per cent	Little clinical significance	
Large 10 per cent	Probably a less differentiated type of squamous-cell carcinoma	Human chorionic gonadotrophin	Painful gynaecomastia	
Adeno- carcinoma 20 per cent	Female prevalence. Develops in lung scars and in fibrosis after exposure to asbestos	Raised CEA		
Alveolar <1 per cent	May be segmental; diffuse or nodular in a lobe or bilateral. Bronchorrhoea a late feature. Metastases few and late			
Adenoma	Hypoglycaemia Carcinoid – flush – wheezing – diarrhoea	Insulin 5 hydroxy- tryptamine Histamine Kallikrein	Raised 5 hydroxyindole Acetic acid	Codeine Bronchodilators Phenoxy-benzamine Serotonin antagonists

The growth of tumours

It is unusual to visualise a bronchial neoplasm less than 1 cm in size. The growth rate of individual tumours varies considerably but it is possible to estimate broadly the rate of cell division or doubling. It is estimated that oat-cell carcinomas double every 30 days, squamous-cell carcinomas every 90 days, and adenocarcinoma every 160 days.

If growth was exponential a single malignant cell would become a 1 mm tumour after its volume had doubled 20 times and a 1 cm tumour mass after 30 doublings. If death were to occur when the primary tumour mass was 5 cm in diameter the duration of life from the onset of growth would be 3.2 years for oat-cell carcinomas, 9.6 years for squamous-cell carcinomas and more than 17 years for adenocarcinomas.

633

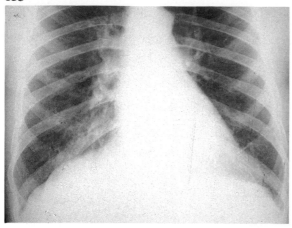

634

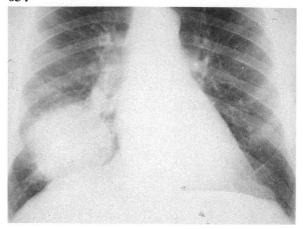

633 and 634   Growth of oat-cell carcinoma. A 58-year-old man presented with haemoptysis and a circular opacity in the right lower lobe. Biopsy revealed oat-cell carcinoma, which is the most rapidly growing histological type. His chest xray was normal two years earlier (**633**).

635

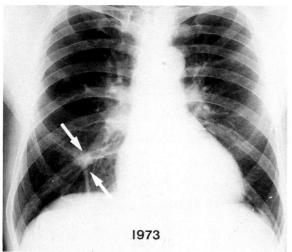

1973

636

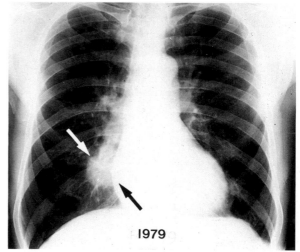

1979

635 and 636   Growth of squamous-cell carcinoma. This elderly bronchitic was found to have a dense circular opacity in the right lower lobe. Numerous sputum specimens revealed squamous carcinoma cells. Regular follow-up films demonstrated slow tumour growth with an increase in diameter of only 2 cm between 1973 and 1979. Fatal cerebral metastases finally developed.

Clinical features and presentation

There are no early or specific symptoms of bronchial carcinoma, but haemoptysis, weight-loss and chest pain are common.

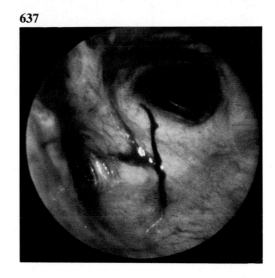

637 Haemoptysis occurs in 70 per cent of patients. Regular daily staining of the sputum is common but massive haemoptysis is rare. Blood is seen lying in the bronchus at fibreoptic bronchoscopy. Cough and shortness of breath may be attributed to smoking and ignored, but haemoptysis and chest pain are seldom neglected.

638

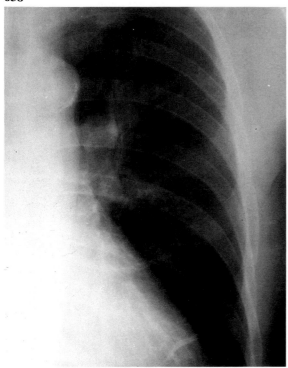

639

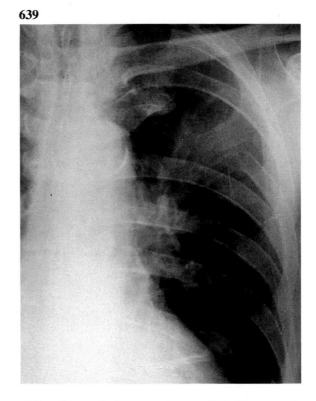

638 Chest pain is a presenting feature in one-third of patients and is frequently mild and poorly localised. This man presented with left pleuritic pain. This initial xray was mistakenly considered normal.

639 Chest pain (same patient as **638**). Four months later the left hilum is more prominent. The fourth left rib is eroded. The histology was squamous-cell carcinoma.

640

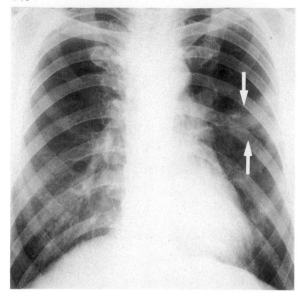

640 Patchy shadowing in the left mid-zone. The patient's symptoms were of left pleurisy and recurrent infections.

641

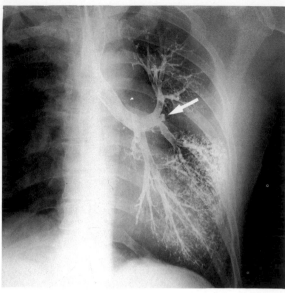

641 Patchy shadowing in the left mid-zone. Bronchogram reveals a block corresponding with this shadow.

Metastases are the presenting features in 10 per cent of patients with bronchial carcinoma.

642

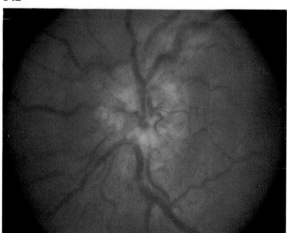

642 Fundus showing papilloedema. Intracranial deposits may present with headache and papilloedema.

643

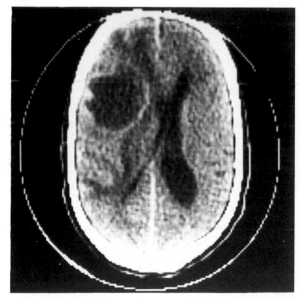

643 Computerised axial tomography (CAT scan) of the skull. A large cystic metastasis occupies the frontal lobe which is displacing the ventricular system. Two other cerebral metastases were demonstrated on different 'cuts'. A small bronchial squamous-cell primary tumour was found at necropsy.

644

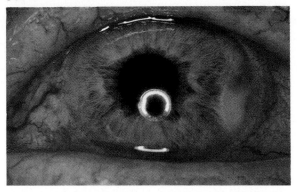

644 Secondary deposit in the iris from squamous bronchial carcinoma. A rare site for a metastasis.

645

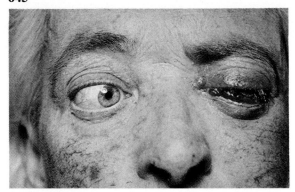

645 Metastasis behind the eye producing external ophthalmoplegia and proptosis.

646

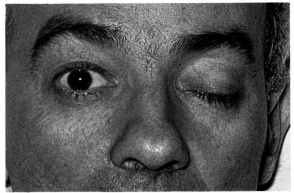

646 Brain-stem lesion resulting in third-nerve palsy. The eye is completely closed, the pupil widely dilated and as all but the superior oblique and lateral rectus are paralysed, the eye points downwards and laterally. This contrasts with partial ptosis which follows interruption of the sympathetic nerve supply.

647

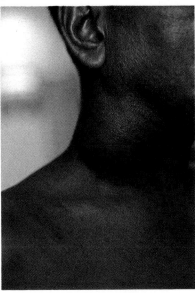

647 Large firm gland in the neck from bronchial carcinoma. This Asian patient had a strongly positive tuberculin test, but he failed to respond to anti-tuberculous chemotherapy. This case demonstrates that not all enlarged neck glands in Asian immigrants are caused by tuberculosis.

648

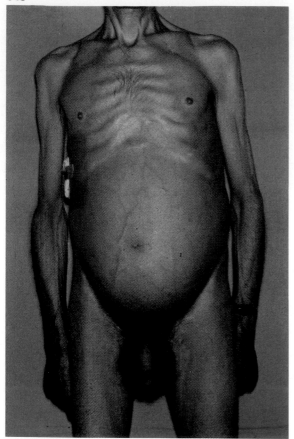

648 Ascites caused by hepatic metastases, from oat-cell carcinoma.

649

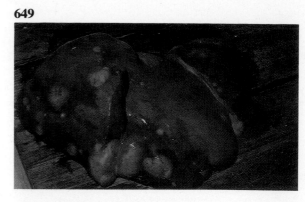

649 Multiple metastases in the liver (necropsy specimen) from oat-cell carcinoma.

650

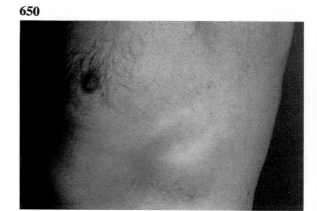

650 Large firm skin metastasis tethered to the ribcage at a site of previous pleural biopsy. The underlying diagnosis was adenocarcinoma.

651

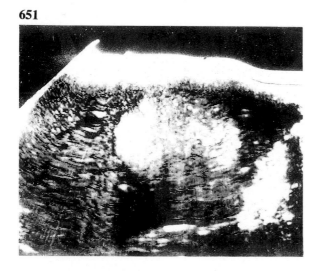

651 Large metastasis in the liver. Parasaggital abdominal ultrasound scan.

652

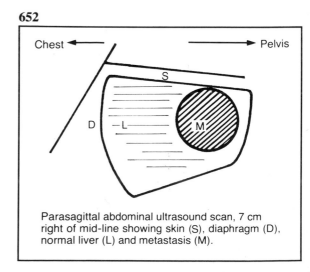

652 Parasaggital abdominal ultrasound scan, 7cm right of midline showing skin (S), diaphragm (D), normal liver (L) and metastasis (M). (Diagram of **651**.)

653

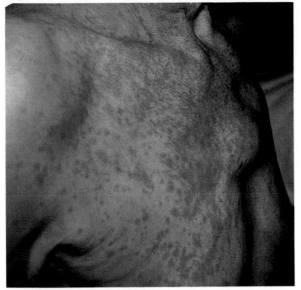

653 Sternal metastases from oat-cell carcinoma. The skin rash is caused by ampicillin sensitivity which developed during treatment for recurrent pneumonia.

654

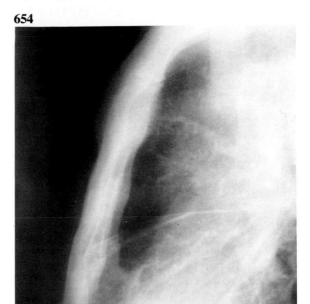

654 Sternal metastases from oat-cell carcinoma. A soft-tissue mass is visible over the sternum. The same patient as **653**.

655

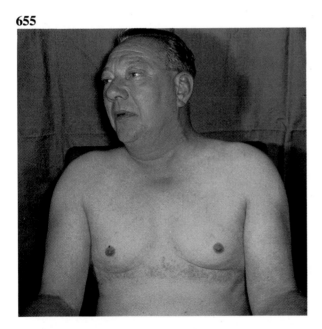

655 Superior vena-caval obstruction in a 53-year-old male who presented with headaches. Note the distended jugular veins, the bloated face, the swollen arms and the dilated veins over the lower chest. The xray shows a large proximal tumour and bronchial biopsy confirmed a squamous-cell carcinoma.

656

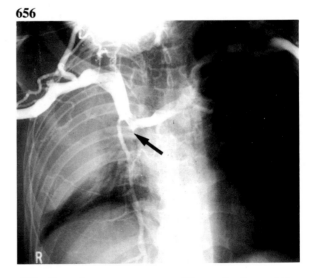

656 Superior vena cavagram. The early phase of this bilateral vena cavagram shows occlusion below the origin of the patent azygos vein (arrowed). (Same patient as **655**.)

Hypertrophic pulmonary osteoarthropathy (HPOA)

This condition is uncommon and painful, and characterised by warm painful swelling of the wrists and ankles usually accompanied by fingernail clubbing. The mechanism by which fingernail clubbing and subperiosteal new-bone formation develop remains unknown, although it is likely that a circulating prosta- glandin-like substance is responsible. Any of the causes of fingernail clubbing may result in HPOA, with the possible exception of con- genital heart disease. Ninety per cent occur with squamous-cell carcinomas while oat-cell carcinomas are only rarely associated with fingernail clubbing or HPOA.

657

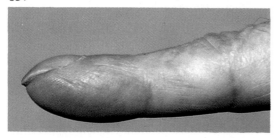

657 Fingernail clubbing. The earliest sign is loss of the angle between the nail and the dorsum of the terminal phalanx caused by hypertrophy of the nailbed tissue.

658

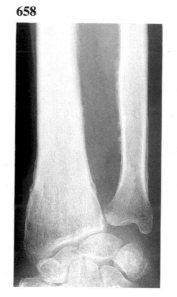

659

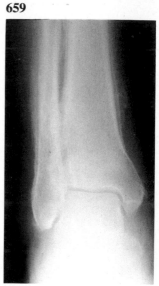

658 Subperiosteal new-bone formation at the wrist.

659 Subperiosteal new-bone formation at the ankle. The 1 mm to 2 mm wide line shadows parallel to the cortex indicate where new bone has been deposited. Effective relief of symptoms with resolution of the radiographic changes fre- quently follows prostaglandin-inhibitor drug therapy.

Table: Causes of fingernail clubbing.

Respiratory
    Bronchial neoplasms – especially squamous-cell
    Pleural tumours
    Bronchiectasis, lung abscess and empyema
    Lung fibrosis – especially asbestosis and cryptogenic fibrosing
    alveolitis

Cardiovascular
    Bacterial endocarditis
    Cyanotic congenital lesions with right to left shunts
    Pulmonary arteriovenous fistula
    Aortic aneurysm

Gastrointestinal
    Cirrhosis

    Chronic diarrhoea ⎯ coeliac disease
    ⎯ ulcerative colitis
    ⎯ Crohn's disease

Familial clubbing

Skin changes in bronchial malignancy

The cutaneous manifestations of malignant tumours in addition to metastatic lesions include changes ranging from non-specific rashes and pigmentation to the following characteristic markers which may precede the underlying cancer by several years.

660

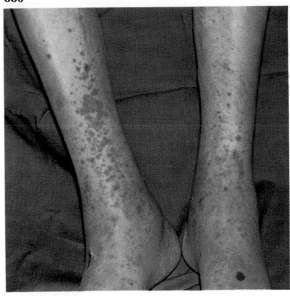

661

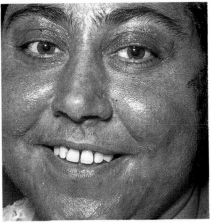

661 Pemphigoid. Large bullae erupt on otherwise normal skin or mucous membranes.

660 Purpura caused by thrombocytopenia. The bone marrow was extensively infiltrated by oat-cell carcinoma.

662

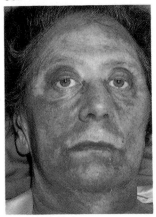

663 Dermatomyositis. Heliotrope markings are present over the finger joints (Gottron's sign). In up to 50 per cent of cases the onset of dermatomyositis in middle-aged adults is associated with a variety of internal neoplasms, including carcinoma of the breast, prostate, intestinal tract and lungs.

663

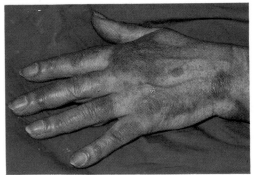

662 Dermatomyositis appears as patchy heliotrope markings on the face and extremities.

664

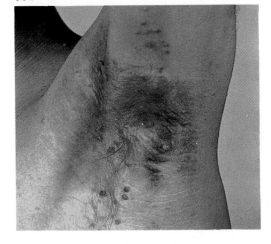

664 Acanthosis nigricans. Symmetrical hyperpigmented hyperkeratotic epidermal changes are found in the flexures. The onset in adult life is frequently associated with intra-abdominal adenocarcinomas. This patient developed a pleural effusion and investigations showed secondary adenocarcinoma infiltrating the pleura.

665 **Herpes zoster** occurs when cell-mediated immunity is impaired and the patient is immunosuppressed by advanced carcinomatosis, reticulosis or lymphatic leukaemia.

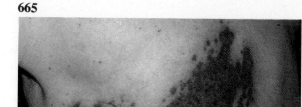

665

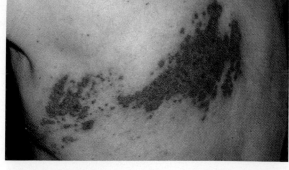

Thoracic inlet tumours (Pancoast)

Tumours lying inconspicuously high at the apex of the lung produce a characteristic clinical picture of severe pain in the arm with weakness of the intrinsic muscles of the hand, Horner's syndrome and hoarseness. Pain is caused by erosion of the upper ribs and involvement of the brachial plexus nerve roots C8, T1. Hoarseness is caused by recurrent laryngeal nerve palsy.

666

1970

666 to 668   Erosion of ribs as a result of Pancoast tumour: 1970 (**666**); 1972 (**667**); 1973 (**668**).

667

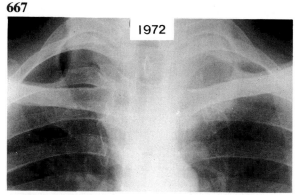

1972

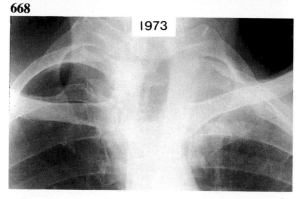

668

1973

669

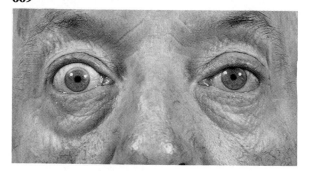

670

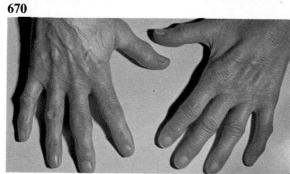

669   Horner's syndrome. Left ptosis and a constricted pupil, caused by involvement of the inferior cervical sympathetic ganglia. The patient volunteered the fact that he does not sweat on the affected side of the face.

670   Brachial plexus nerve root infiltration. The small muscles of the hand and thenar eminence show gross wasting. This is caused by infiltration of the left C8, T1 nerve roots and disuse atrophy.

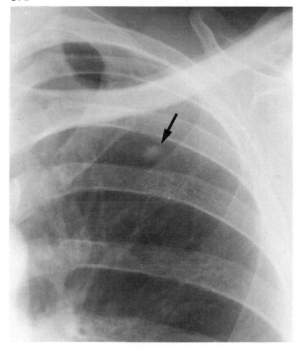

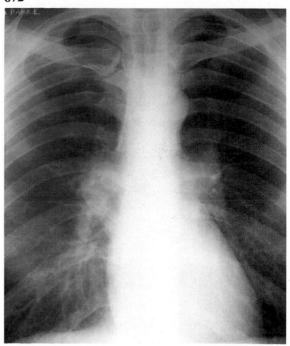

671 **Early bronchial carcinomas** are usually found by chance. This patient had a very small circular lesion (arrowed). At thoracotomy a small adenocarcinoma was removed. The average size of a peripheral tumour is 3 cm at the time of diagnosis.

672 **The right hilum appears abnormally dense** on the PA film taken after a minor haemoptysis. Fibreoptic bronchoscopy showed a tumour adjacent to the middle-lobe bronchus. The histology was squamous-cell carcinoma.

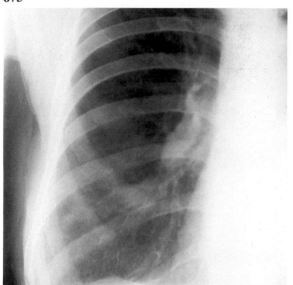

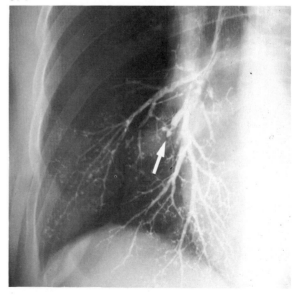

673 **Recurrent right lower-lobe pneumonia.** Chest infections may fail to resolve or may recur as in this patient. Note the consolidated segment.

674 **Bronchogram showing occlusion of the posterior basal bronchus by tumour (arrowed).** A squamous-cell tumour was successfully resected. (Same patient as **673**.)

The radiographic appearances are variable. Peripheral carcinomas appear as rounded lesions which may have 'pseudopodia' radiating from the surface. Central tumours are likely to cause collapse or consolidation of a lobe or segment, or involve hilar and mediastinal glands which enlarge. Effusions are common and diaphragmatic paralysis caused by mediastinal entrapment of the phrenic nerve may occur. Necrosis in a carcinoma mimics the radiographic appearances of a lung abscess.

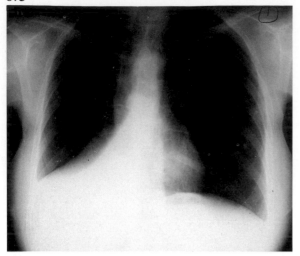

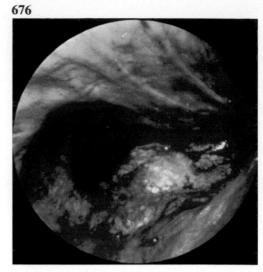

675 Proximal oat-cell carcinoma caused collapse of right lower lobe. Within one month the right lung totally collapsed.

676 Carcinoma in right main bronchus responsible for collapse in right lower lobe of **675**. The main carina is widened by adjacent malignant glands.

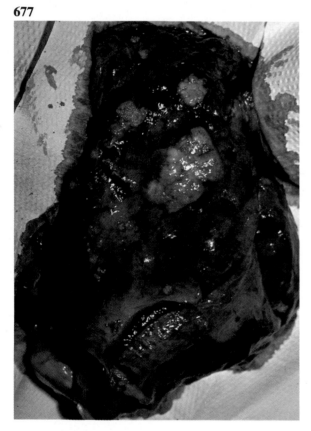

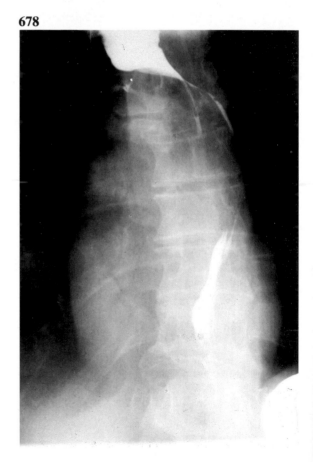

677 Multiple pleural metastases were the source of blood-stained pleural effusion.

678 Barium swallow showing considerable deviation of the oesophagus caused by enlarged mediastinal glands. Dysphagia may occur with proximal tumours, as a result of extrinsic pressure upon the oesophagus from enlarged glands or stenosis occurring with direct infiltration into the oesophageal wall by tumour.

679

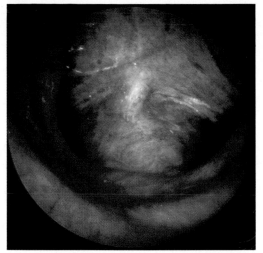

679 Bronchoscopy shows widened carina caused by enlarged mediastinal glands (*see* page 38).

680 Tracheo-oesophageal fistula. Seventy-five per cent of bronchial carcinomas arise centrally so they are often inoperable. This oat-cell carcinoma invaded the oesophagus which then perforated during a course of palliative radiotherapy. Note the fistula (arrowed) and the right main bronchus outlined by contrast medium. (*Gastrograffin oesophageal contrast study.*)

680

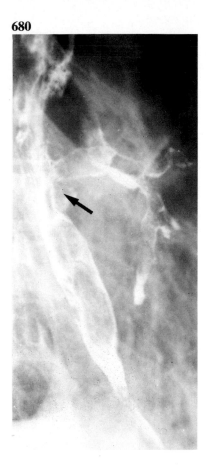

Squamous-cell carcinoma

681

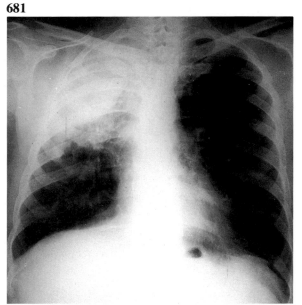

682

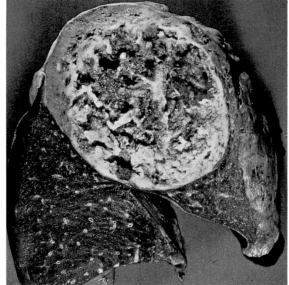

681 and 682 Squamous-cell carcinoma involving the right upper lobe which presented with pain and haemoptysis. The xray showed a dense right upper-lobe opacity. A pneumonectomy was performed and the specimen showed a cavitating necrotic tumour. The yellow granular 'cheesy' appearance is typical of a squamous-cell carcinoma. Obstruction by either intra-luminal growth or by stenosing tumour encircling the wall may lead to infection and collapse of the lung distal to the lesion.

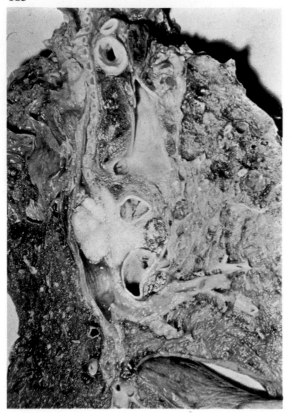

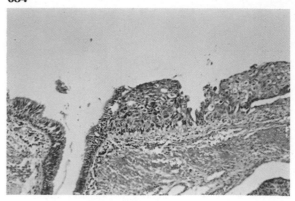

684 Squamous cell carcinoma. Operative specimen showing malignant change in the bronchial epithelium. Note the characteristic intercellular bridges, cell nest formation, keratin and whorling arrangement of polygonal neoplastic epithelial cells.

685

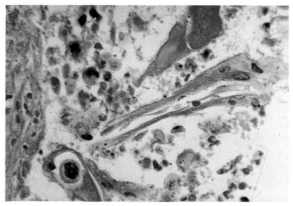

683 A squamous-cell carcinoma occludes the left upper-lobe bronchus, and distal to it is fibrosis and infection.

685 Squamous-cell carcinoma. Bronchial biopsy specimen. The bronchial mucosa (not shown) was normal. Exfoliated tumour cells lie in the bronchial lumen. *(H&E ×60)*

686

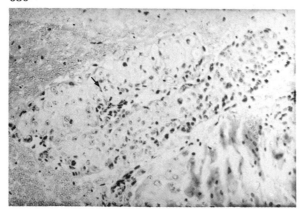

687

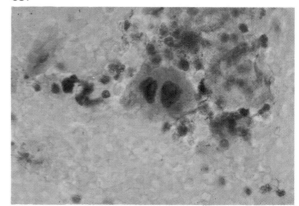

686 Aspiration percutaneous needle biopsy specimen. A group of polygonal squamous neoplastic cells are present (arrowed) within surrounding bloodclot.

687 Squamous-cell carcinoma. Sputum cytology. Cells occurring singly and of variable size are most common with irregular nuclei and eosinophilic cytoplasm. Multinucleated cells may be found.

688

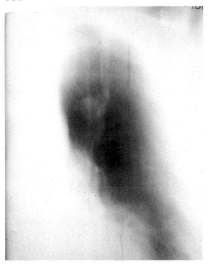

688 Well defined circular opacity lying in left upper lobe (tomographic view).

Small-cell carcinoma (oat-cell)

Small-cell carcinoma commonly arises in major bronchi and then spreads rapidly to the regional lymphatics. The pulmonary vessels are involved at an early stage and widespread haematogenous metastases are frequent at presentation. Most bronchial carcinomas occurring in patients under 40 years of age are of this type.

690 Oat-cell carcinoma accounts for about one-fifth of bronchial carcinomas. These highly malignant tumours frequently arise in major bronchi and show a tendency for early lymphatic spread to the regional lymph nodes. In this case the tumour has arisen in the apical segment of the left lower lobe spreading to the hilar glands and to the pleura. Blood-borne metastases occur early.

691 and 692 Pyopneumothorax, secondary to oat-cell carcinoma of the bronchus. This patient presented with a pyopneumothorax caused by pus and air escaping into the pleural space after rupture of a lung abscess.

689

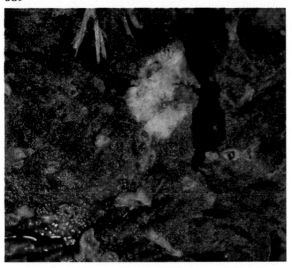

689 Lobectomy specimen of a 1 cm squamous-cell carcinoma. The tumour has been bisected. Resection is curative at this early stage if secondary spread has not occurred.

690

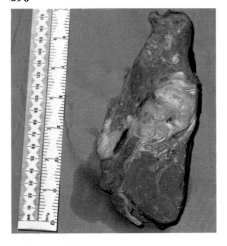

691

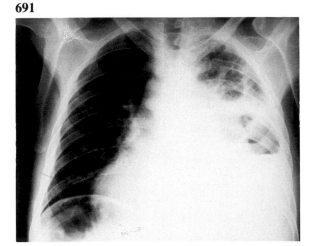

692

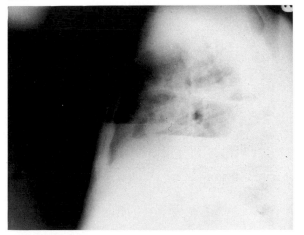

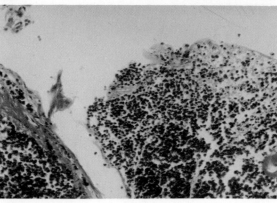

693 Oat-cell carcinoma. Bronchial biopsy. The cells are small with deeply staining nuclei and scanty cytoplasm and although of various shapes, tend to be spherical or oat shaped. Oat-cell carcinomas were regarded as arising from the germinal layer of cells in the bronchial epithelium, but are now known to arise from the Kulchitsky-like cells lying in both the bronchial epithelium and mucous glands; they therefore share some features of bronchial carcinoid tumours.

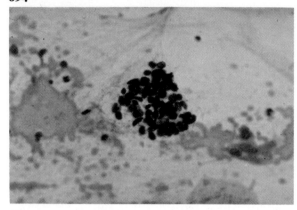

694 Oat-cell carcinoma. Brush biopsy, showing characteristic clumps of dark-staining cells.

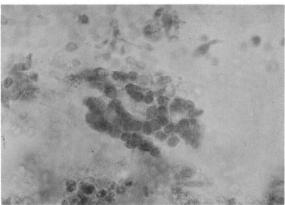

695 Oat-cell carcinoma. Sputum cytology. Clumps of dark-staining cells. Each nucleus contains one or two nucleoli.

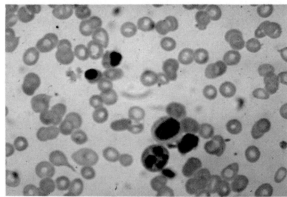

696 Leucoerythroblastic anaemia. Normoblasts in peripheral blood film suggest bone-marrow infiltration by malignant cells.

697

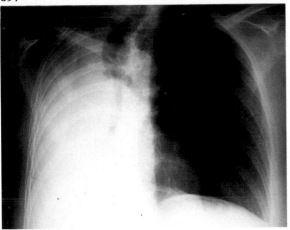

697 Oat-cell carcinoma occluding right main bronchus with collapse of the lung.

698

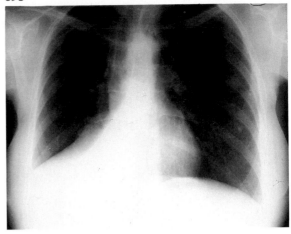

698 Oat-cell carcinoma. Radiotherapy rapidly reduced the tumour bulk with re-expansion of the upper and middle lobe. Oat-cell carcinomas are very sensitive to radiotherapy and cytotoxic drugs, particularly cyclophosphamide, methotrexate, doxorubicin, vincristine, lomustine and procarbazine. (Same patient as in **697**.)

699

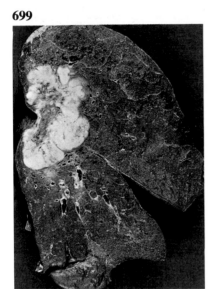

Adenocarcinoma

699 Adenocarcinoma. Whole lung section. Most glandular carcinomas arise in the periphery of the lung. Growth is usually slow and a large size may be reached before symptoms occur. Adenocarcinoma accounts for about one-fifth of bronchial carcinomas. The tumour arises from mucous glands in small bronchi at the lung periphery. Tumours arising in lung scars caused by asbestosis or healed tuberculosis or chronic interstitial fibrosis are most often of this type. No clear association between adenocarcinoma and cigarette smoking has been established.

700

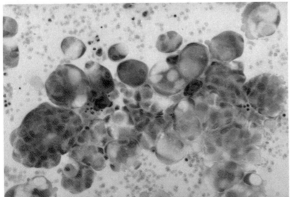

700 Cytological smear of pleural fluid showing adeno-carcinoma cells. Considerable experience is required to diagnose correctly the presence of malignant cells in pleural fluid.

701

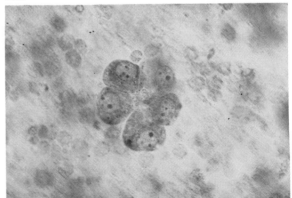

701 Sputum smear showing a cluster of adeno-carcinoma cells. The distinctive features are the ample vacuolated cytoplasm and multiple nucleoli.

Large-cell carcinoma

These poorly differentiated tumours arise from squamous epithelium. Growth is rapid with widespread haematogenous dissemination reminiscent of small-cell carcinoma.

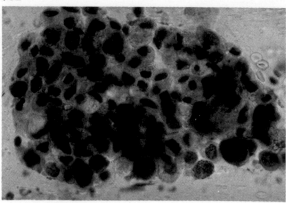

702 Large-cell carcinoma. Aspiration biopsy specimen showing darkly staining medium and large cells.

Alveolar-cell carcinoma

Alveolar-cell carcinoma accounts for less than one per cent of all malignant intrathoracic tumours.

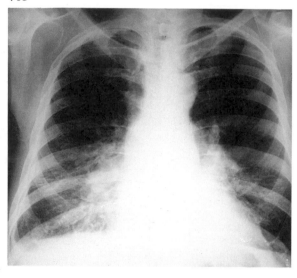

703 Alveolar-cell carcinoma. Bilateral lower zone shadowing was initially attributed to chronic pulmonary oedema in this emphysematous patient.

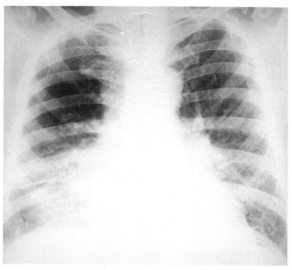

704 Alveolar-cell carcinoma. Three months later more extensive shadowing is visible. A tissue diagnosis was established by trephine biopsy.

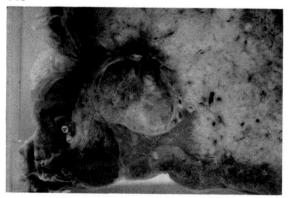

705 Alveolar-cell carcinoma. Macroscopic specimen showing a chronic abscess cavity and adjacent lung consolidated with greyish-white tumour.

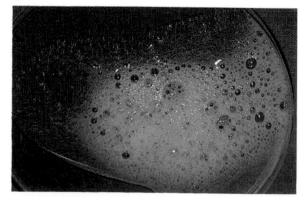

706 Alveolar-cell carcinoma. Bronchorrhoea is a common but not invariable feature. The sputum was copious and frothy.

Secondary tumours in the lung

Pulmonary metastases may be found in about one-third of all cases of malignant disease, some three-quarters of which originate in the breast, bones, urogenital or gastrointestinal tract. Spread to the lungs is by the vascular or lymphatic systems.

The common radiographic appearance of pulmonary metastases may be:

1 Discrete and usually rounded, single or multiple 'cannon-ball' opacities.
2 A widespread 'snowstorm' pattern.
3 Coarse linear shadowing caused by lymphatic spread.

Pain from pleural involvement and dyspnoea caused by extensive embolic small-vessel occlusion may occur.

707

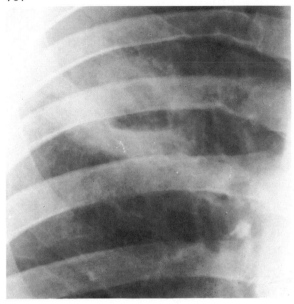

708

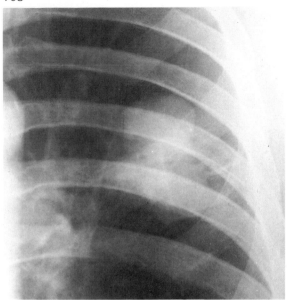

707 and 708 Hypernephroma. A single lobulated mass in the left lung and a cavitating thick-walled shadow in the right lung were caused by metastases from hypernephroma. It is unusual for metastases to cavitate but when they do hypernephroma is often the cause.

709

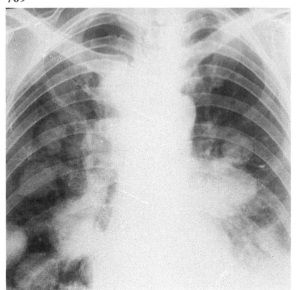

710

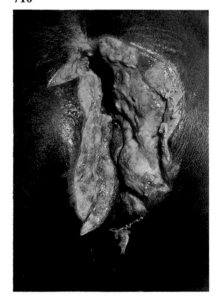

709 and 710 Multiple 'cannon ball' shadows together with a left pleural effusion from a large ulcerating rectal carcinoma.

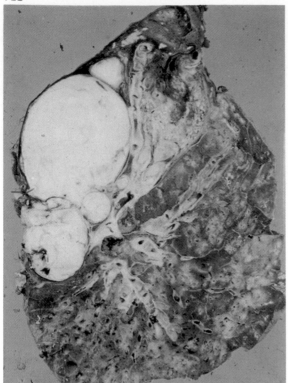

711 Multiple secondary deposits from carcinoma of the colon. The lower lobe contains multiple small deposits, whereas the upper lobe contains large tumour masses. Carcinoembryonic antigen was strongly positive.

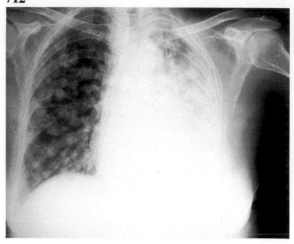

712 Multiple secondary deposits with left pleural effusion from a seminoma.

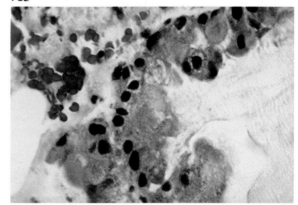

713 Pleural biopsy with mucus-secreting cells from metastasis.

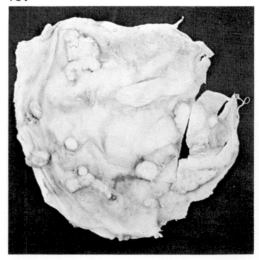

714 The pleura shows multiple yellow secondary deposits.

715 Metastatic adenocarcinoma in the lung. The primary site was not identified in this patient. Most cases arise from gynaecological, prostatic or breast primary tumours. This group of malignant tumours can be palliated by chemotherapy, therefore a detailed search for the primary site can be worthwhile.

Other possible primary sites include occult primary tumours of the pancreas, stomach, colon, liver or lung.

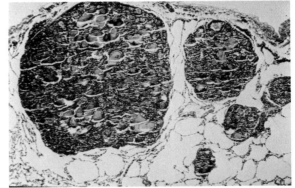

716

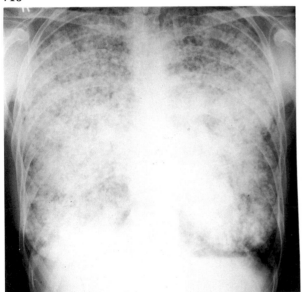

717

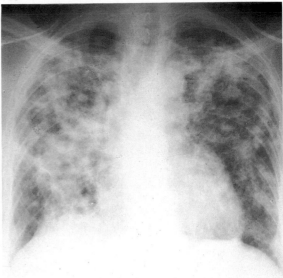

717 Metastatic follicular thyroid carcinoma. Same patient as **716**. Colloid containing thyroid tissue together with lung is seen in this drill biopsy specimen.

716 Disseminated haematogenous metastases from a thyroid carcinoma. This 'snowstorm' of metastatic deposits remained unchanged for many months because of the slow growth of the tumour. The initial radiographic appearance was of a fine micronodular pattern.

Similar appearances are seen in pulmonary metastases arising from other highly vascular primary tumours, such as chorion carcinoma, osteosarcoma and renal carcinoma.

718

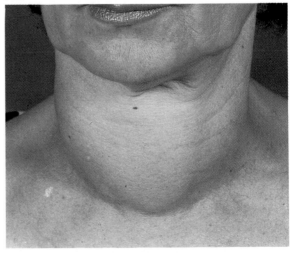

718 Multinodular goitre which underwent malignant change: same patient as **716**.

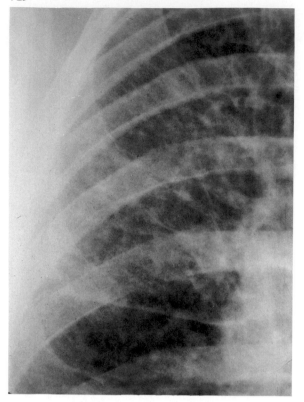

719 Long-hair line 'shadows' in the upper lung fields running from the hilum towards the periphery. These lines (Kerley-A lines) represent lymphatics infiltrated by tumour. This appearance is a radiographic manifestation of lymphangitis carcinomatosa.

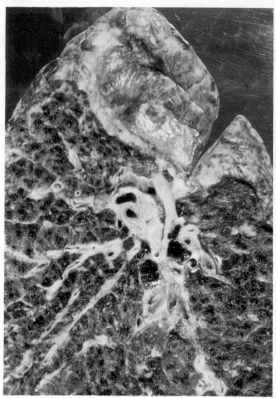

720 Lymphangitis carcinomatosa. Cut surface of the lung. The walls of small bronchi and lymphatic vessels are infiltrated by tumour.

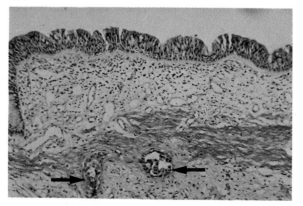

721 Lymphangitis carcinomatosa showing secondary carcinoma cells filling the perivascular lymphatics. *(H&E ×40)*

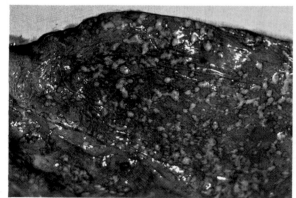

722 Malignant infiltration of the pleura.

Bronchial adenomas

Bronchial adenomas usually present at a much earlier age than carcinomas, often before the fifth decade. Cough and haemoptysis with signs of lobar collapse are common.

723

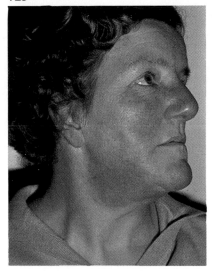

Adenomas are derived from the duct epithelium of bronchial mucous glands. About 90 per cent of these tumours are carcinoids, the remainder resemble salivary gland tumours.

724

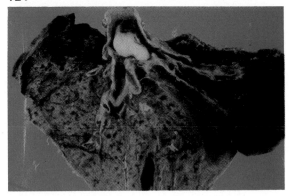

724 Whole lung section of bronchial carcinoid occluding a lobar bronchus. Local excision may be sufficient although some carcinoids metastasise to lymph nodes, liver or bone.

723 Carcinoid facial flushing. This dramatic sign is rare in bronchial carcinoids but common in gut carcinoids. Abdominal cramp, diarrhoea, oedema, wheeze, breathlessness and flushing are caused by those tumours releasing various vasoactive substances. The release of these substances from a primary lung carcinoid may damage valves in the left side of the heart. These vasoactive substances include 5 hydroxytryptamine, histamine, prostaglandins and kallikrein. In addition adenomas may secrete insulin causing hypoglycaemia.

725 Carcinoid tumour. Bronchoscopy provides confirmatory histology in 75 per cent of cases. Beware, carcinoid tumour can readily be confused with oat-cell carcinoma.

725

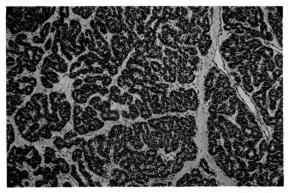

726

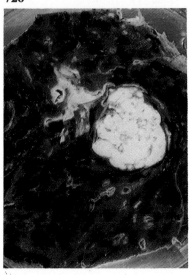

Hamartoma

726 Hamartoma. Foci of calcification are present in the solitary well-circumscribed lobulated creamy-white mass. Hamartomas contain the normal tissues of the bronchial wall with cartilage mixed connective tissue and gland-like clefts lined by cuboidal epithelium. It is often solitary, subpleural and a chance finding during routine chest xray. It may 'bounce off' the end of an aspiration biopsy needle because it is so hard.

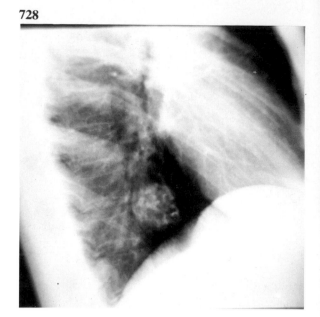

727 and 728 Hamartoma. The PA film shows an abnormal contour to the right diaphragm. The lateral film shows a solitary sharply demarcated round lesion in which speckles of 'popcorn' calcification are present.

Hodgkin's disease

Hodgkin's disease is characterised by painless and progressive lymphadenopathy with cachexia, anaemia, pruritis and fever.

Mediastinal gland involvement is common. Primary disease of the lung is rare.

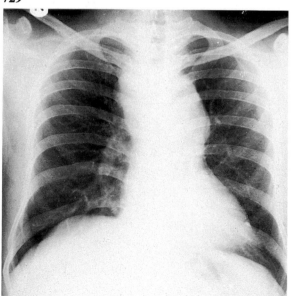

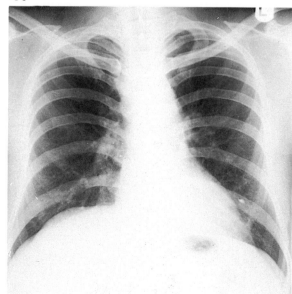

729 and 730 Hodgkin's disease. Xray showing enlarged mediastinal lymph nodes. No evidence of the disease was present below the diaphragm so it remained stage 2 disease and suitable for radiotherapy. Radiotherapy caused rapid shrinkage of the mediastinal lymphadenopathy (**730**).

731

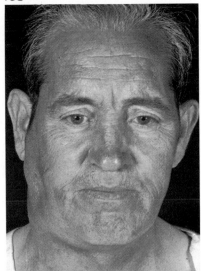

731 Hodgkin's disease. Large lymph nodes on both sides of the neck. There was also enlargement of the mediastinal lymph nodes. (Same patient as **729**.)

732

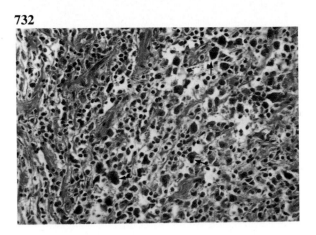

732 Hodgkin's disease. Lymph node histology. The tumour is composed of histiocytes, polymorphs and Reed–Sternberg giant cells (arrowed) with 'mirror image' double nuclei.

733

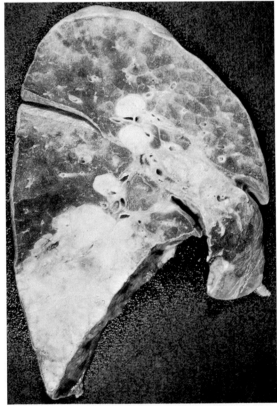

733 Primary Hodgkin's disease of the lung may occasionally arise in the lymph nodes related to bronchi. Macroscopically the surface of the tumour is yellow and lobulated. The lower and middle lobes are involved and separate nodules are present in the upper lobe.

734

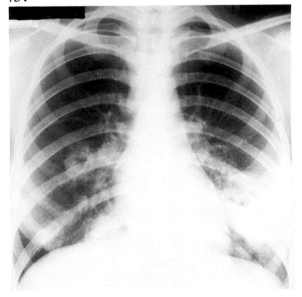

734 Cavitating Hodgkin's disease. Coarse well-defined nodules may cavitate or become confluent. Cough, chest pain, fever and pruritis were the presenting symptoms. Diagnosis was only made from specimens obtained at thoracotomy.

24 Bronchiectasis

The term bronchiectasis describes abnormal dilation of the bronchi, but in general usage it also implies bronchial-wall destruction. Saccular bronchiectasis is the classic form characterised by irregular dilatations and narrowings. The term cystic is used when the dilatations are especially large and numerous. Drainage of secretions from the involved bronchi is impaired resulting in chronic infection of the affected lobe or segment. The principal clinical feature is a chronic cough productive of copious, often blood-stained, sputum. The physical signs include cyanosis and coarse crackles with wheeze.

In advanced cases chronic malnutrition, sinusitis, finger clubbing (*see* page 230), cor pulmonale and frequent bronchopulmonary infections may occur. Advanced bronchiectasis is often accompanied by hypertrophy and anastomoses between the bronchial and pulmonary vessels, causing right to left shunts which are the site of haemoptysis. Haemoptysis may be severe.

Whatever the initial cause, inflammation damages the bronchial walls leading to replacement of normal ciliated cuboidal epithelium.

Bronchiectasis usually is acquired in childhood, often after a recognisable respiratory infection complicating measles, pertussis, influenza or after repeated or prolonged pneumonitis. See below for a classification of bronchiectasis.

Table: Causes of bronchiectasis.

Congenital	Kartagener's syndrome
	Bronchial mucocele
	Sequestrated segment
	Cystic fibrosis
	Hypogammaglobulinaemia
Acquired	Obstruction of small bronchi
	Measles or whooping cough
	Pneumonia
	Bronchiolitis in infancy
	Postprimary tuberculosis damaging upper lobe
	'Middle-lobe' syndrome in tuberculosis
	Proximal bronchiectasis in asthmatic with pulmonary eosinophilia

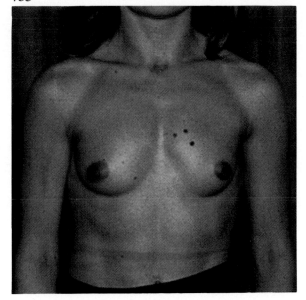

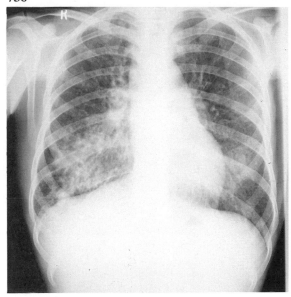

735 and 736 Generalised bronchiectasis. This 26-year-old woman developed bronchiectasis after severe infantile whooping cough. About 50 ml of purulent sputum was expectorated daily. Tracheostomy was performed during a life-threatening infection at 21 years of age, and since then cyanosis and finger clubbing had developed. Exercise tolerance was limited to 100 yards on flat ground.

Note the hyperinflated 'square-shaped' chest and powerful intercostal muscles which are a consequence of long-standing airflow obstruction.

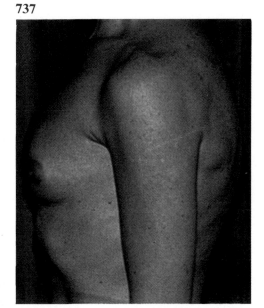

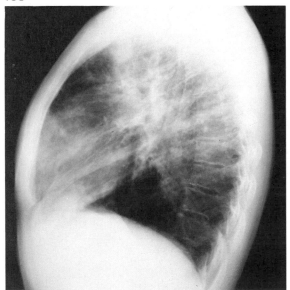

737 and 738 Generalised bronchiectasis (lateral view). Note the deep posteroanterior depth of the chest. The xrays (**736** and **738**) show 'tramline' shadows most prominent in the right lower zone.

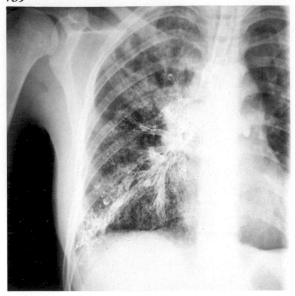

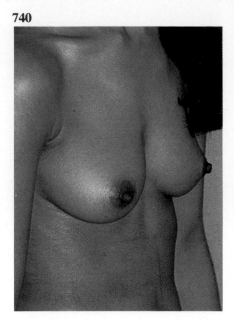

739 Bronchogram showing dilated bronchi with cystic changes involving the right lower lobe. (Same patient as **735**.)

740 Unilateral bronchiectasis. Flattening of the right side of the chest in long-standing unilateral bronchiectasis of unknown cause.

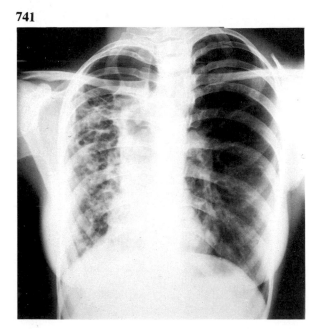

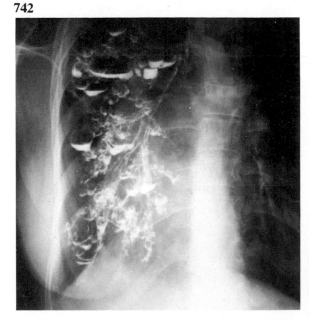

741 Bronchiectasis. Contracted destroyed right lung with many cystic spaces. The mediastinum is deviated to the affected side and the rib space is narrowed showing the marked loss of volume. (Same patient as **740**.)

742 Bronchiectasis. Bronchogram showing large cystic spaces and distortion of the normal right bronchial tree.

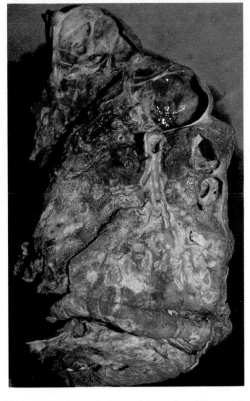

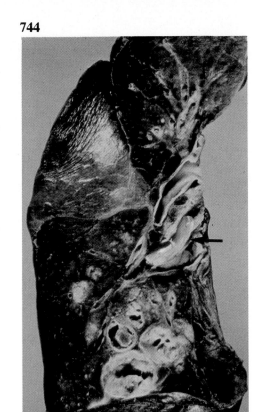

743 Widespread bronchiectasis. The right pneumonectomy specimen showing widespread bronchiectasis with large cystic spaces in the upper lobe,
considerable destruction of the lung substance and a
thick mantle of inflammatory tissue surrounding the
walls of dilated bronchi in lower lobe. The lung was
functionless and the major source of sputum. Symptoms
were much improved after surgery. (Same patient as
740 to 742.)

744 Bronchiectasis. Broken dentures can be
hazardous. This large fragment was inhaled during
sleep. Infection developed distal to the obstruction
destroying the bronchi and leaving large cystic spaces.

745

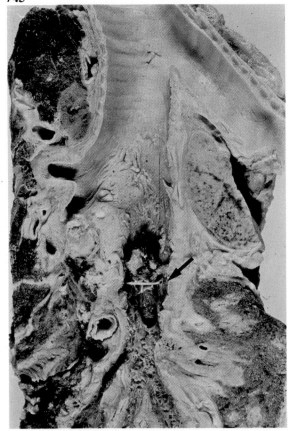

745 Bronchiectasis. Bronchial obstruction may contribute to bronchiectasis. A rabbit vertebra was inhaled
and impacted in the lower lobe bronchus. Infection
occurred beyond this obstruction with dilatation,
infection and destruction of the bronchial walls.

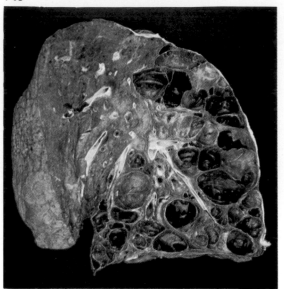

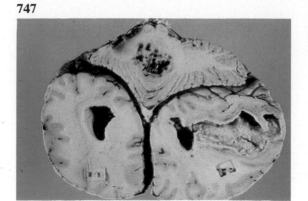

747 Fatal cerebral metastatic abscess. A rare event since the introduction of antibiotics.

746 Extensive cystic bronchiectasis in necropsy specimen. Death occurred from a cerebral abscess.

748

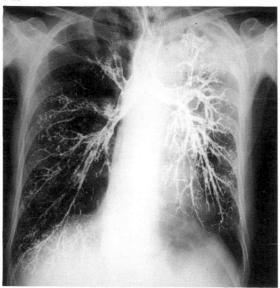

748 Upper-lobe bronchiectasis is almost always due to healed apical pulmonary tuberculosis.

749

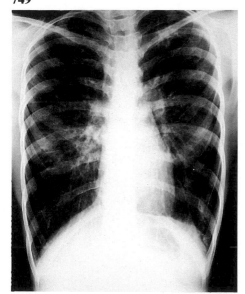

749 Cystic fibrosis with bronchiectasis and hyper-inflation. This is an autosomal recessive disorder characterised by hypertrophy of mucus-secreting glands, a high sweat sodium chloride concentration and exocrine pancreatic insufficiency causing malabsorption and failure of growth. The incidence of asymptomatic heterozygotic carriers is 1 in 25 live births and of homozygotes is 1 in 2500 live births.

Lung function is progressively impaired. Infection with S. aureus in childhood and P. aeruginosa in adult life, pneumothorax, haemoptysis, nasal polyps and male infertility are common problems.

25 Miscellaneous disorders

Kartagener's immotile cilia syndrome

There is a generalised congenital ciliary immotility (*see* Table). Poor mucociliary transport in the respiratory system results in rhinitis, sinusitis, recurrent bronchitis and bronchiectasis. Immotility of spermatozoa causes male infertility. When the rotation of the embryonic gut is not guided by ciliary movements, the rotation will take place at random resulting in situs inversus in about one-half of affected individuals. This syndrome is far commoner than we realise. The chest physician should arrange for sperm examination of infertile males with recurrent bronchitis, even in the absence of situs inversus.

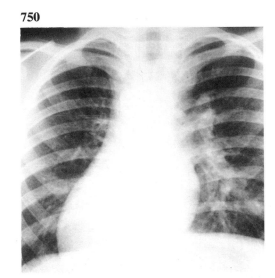

750

750   Dextrocardia.

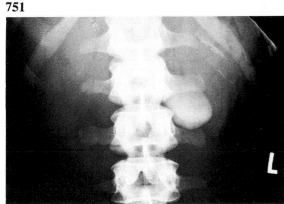

751

751   Cholecystogram demonstrates a left-sided gall bladder.

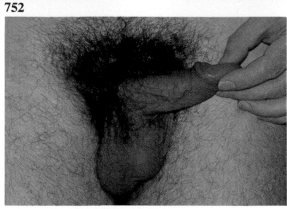

752

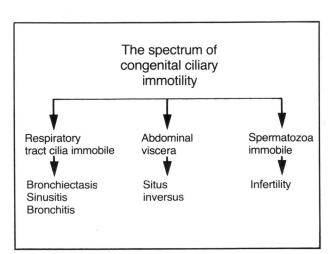

```
The spectrum of
congenital ciliary
immotility

Respiratory          Abdominal          Spermatozoa
tract cilia immobile viscera            immobile

Bronchiectasis       Situs              Infertility
Sinusitis            inversus
Bronchitis
```

752   Dextrocardia – a sign. Whereas the left testis normally hangs lower than the right, this situation is reversed in situs inversus. This may be regarded as a bizarre physical sign of dextrocardia.

753

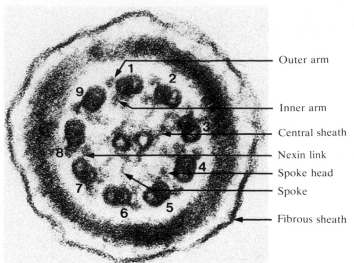

753 **Micrograph giving definition of terms used for various components of sperm flagellum** ×320,000. The spermatozoa of men with this syndrome are immotile but living. The sperm tails have flagellar mutants in which sperm axonemes lack dynein arms or spoke heads.

754

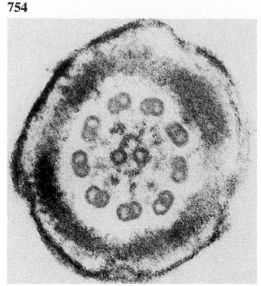

754 **Immotile spermatozoa with absent dynein arms.**

Alveolar proteinosis

Lipoproteinaceous material is deposited in the distal air sacs with impairment of gas exchange.

755

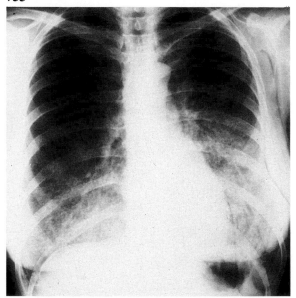

755 **Alveolar proteinosis.** Fever is followed by progressive dyspnoea, chest pain and cough. The physical signs are minimal compared with the radiological changes which simulate pulmonary oedema.

756

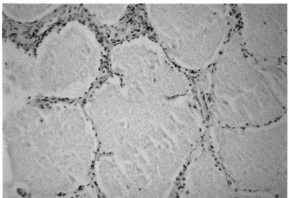

756 **Alveolar proteinosis.** The alveoli contain granular eosinophilic exudate which is strongly positive to periodic-acid-Schiff (PAS) staining, and also stains heavily for lipid. Considerable improvement followed bronchial lavage, but deterioration and death as a result of respiratory failure or infection is the usual outcome. Alveolar macrophages are lipid-rich and stain PAS positive. They contain lamellar inclusions of whorls of lipoproteinaceous material filling the cytoplasm of the macrophage. These macrophages provide poor defence against such exotic infections as nocardiosis to which these patients are peculiarly susceptible (*see* Tables on pages 123 and 124).

Pulmonary arteriovenous fistula

This abnormality is caused by the persistence of foetal capillary anastomoses between the pulmonary arteries and veins. In about one-fifth of cases the lesions are multiple and similar lesions may develop in other organs. About half are associated with hereditary haemorrhagic telangiectasia.

Dyspnoea, cyanosis, polycythaemia and finger clubbing are features of major right to left shunts of deoxygenated blood.

757

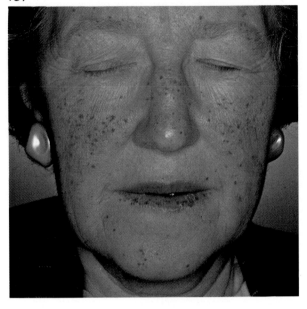

758

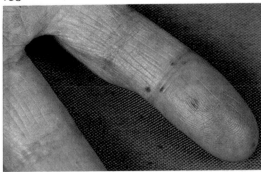

757 and 758   Pulmonary arteriovenous fistula. A florid example of hereditary haemorrhagic telangiectasia (Osler–Rendu disease).

Telangiectasia of the lips and finger gave helpful clues in diagnosing the cause of this patient's haemoptysis.

759

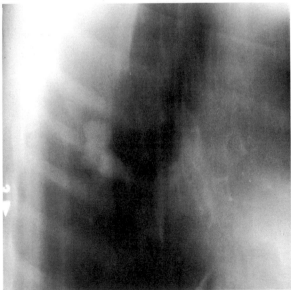

759   Tomogram showing a lobulated opacity in a patient presenting with haemoptysis.

760

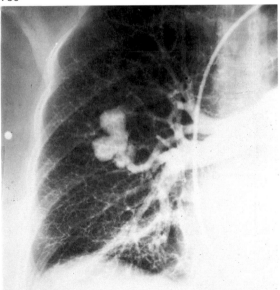

760   Pulmonary artery angiogram demonstrating an arteriovenous fistula: same patient as 757 and 759.

Idiopathic mediastinal fibrosis

A rare disorder of unknown aetiology causing progressive fibrosis of the mediastinal tissues. with compression of the vena cava, oesophagus and trachea.

The onset is usually in middle-age with dyspnoea or superior vena-caval obstruction.

761

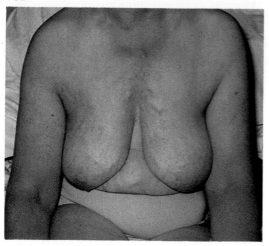

761 Idiopathic mediastinal fibrosis causes superior vena-caval obstruction. Note the swollen arms and the tortuous collaterals over the anterior chest, which had remained unchanged for five years.

762

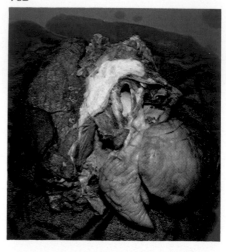

762 Macroscopic specimen. The upper mediastinum is infiltrated with dense fibrous tissue which has strangled the superior vena cava, the right pulmonary artery and hilum. The superior vena cava is stenotic and only admitted a 1mm probe. The right pulmonary artery is narrowed by extrinsic compression.

763

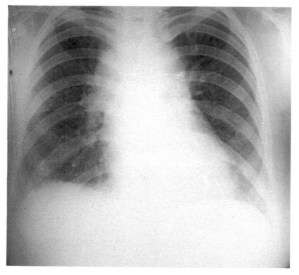

763 Mediastinal widening in idiopathic mediastinal fibrosis. A middle-aged woman who presented with breathlessness and superior vena-caval obstruction.

764

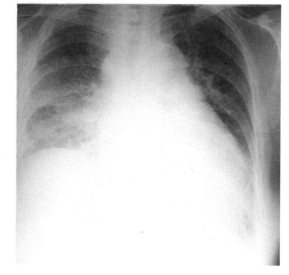

764 Mediastinal widening. Same patient as **763** after 15 years. The right lung has contracted and the mediastinum widened. The clinical appearance is shown in **761**.

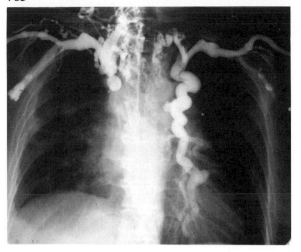

765 Superior vena cavogram. The early film shows no dye in the superior vena cava and gross dilatation of vessels to the left of the mediastinum.

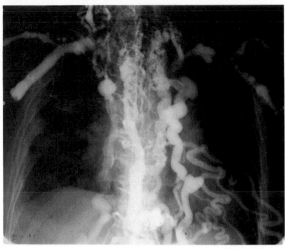

766 Superior vena cavogram. The late film shows some dye has reached the inferior vena cava. Flow in the superior vena cava is reduced to a trickle.

Pulmonary alveolar microlithiasis

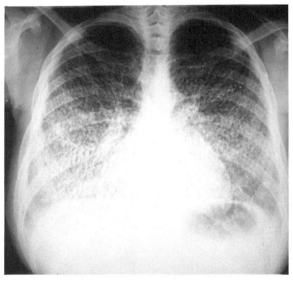

767 Pulmonary alveolar microlithiasis is often familial. The radiograph appearance is of dense widespread miliary mottling with a predominance of lowerlobe shadowing. This mottling represents extensive intra-alveolar deposits of calcium-containing bodies.

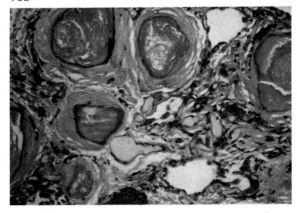

768 Histology. Multiple intra-alveolar calcospherites with concentric laminations giving rise to an 'onionskin' appearance. The alveolar walls become damaged. At necropsy the lungs are remarkable for their weight and hardness. Pulmonary alveolar microlithiasis may be associated with mitral stenosis. Most cases are idiopathic and show a familial tendency. Symptoms may be absent in spite of extensive radiographic shadowing but cough, dyspnoea and respiratory failure eventually supervene. *(PAS stain ×130).*

769

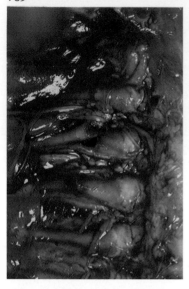

769 Fractured neck of ribs which may occur when an infant's chest is forcibly squeezed by an adult; in this case a battered child.

770

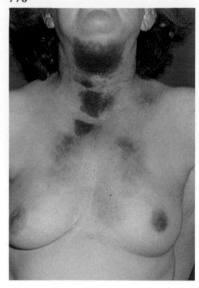

770 Bruising over the neck and anterior chest with fracture of three ribs shown in xray. Victim of road traffic accident.

771

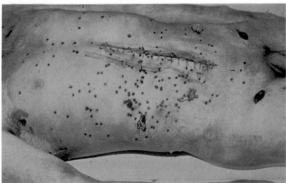

771 Gamekeepers' occupational hazard. He was accidentally shot by an inexperienced shooting party.

772

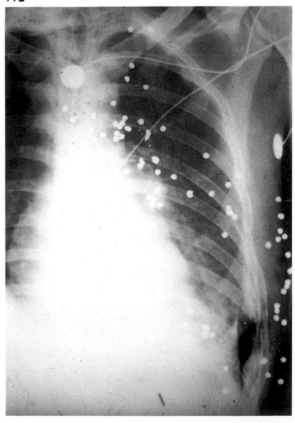

772 Chest xray shows gunshot pellets, pneumothorax and fractured ribs.

773

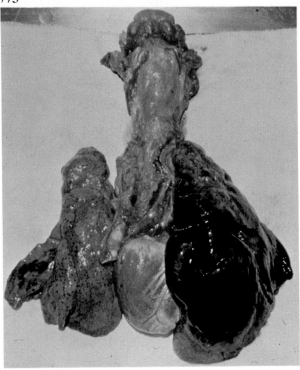

773 Fatal pulmonary contusion caused by blast injury. The left lung is oedematous and suffused with blood.

774

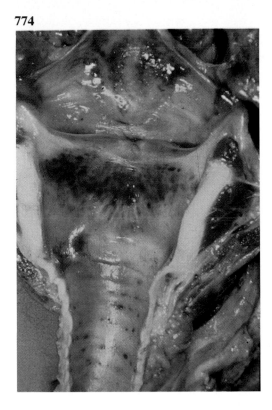

774 Laryngeal ecchymoses after blast injury.

Cervical ribs

775

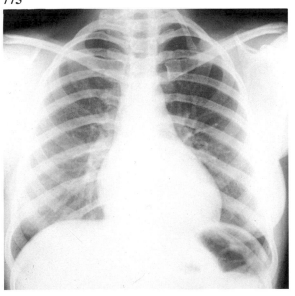

775 Cervical rib. Symptoms, caused by compression of a nerve or blood vessel, occur in 10 per cent of patients. Note the hypertransradiancy resulting from the right mastectomy.

776

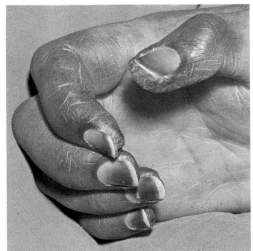

776 Subclavian artery compression causes digital ischaemia. At operation dense fibrous tissue arising from the rib was encircling the artery.

Erythema multiforme
(Stevens–Johnson syndrome)

Erythema multiforme is a systemic hypersensitivity vasculitis, provoked by virus infections, Mycoplasma pneumoniae, vaccination, and drugs (sulphonamides, barbiturates, aspirin, and sulphonylurea drugs).

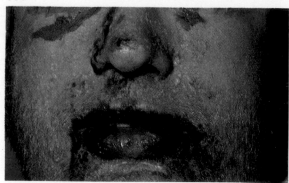

777 Widespread bullous eruptions, particularly involving mucocutaneous junctions are evident. The chest xray may show pneumonia, miliary or nodular shadows, resolving as the skin lesions heal.

The scimitar syndrome

Anomalous pulmonary venous drainage of the right lung to the inferior vena cava.

778

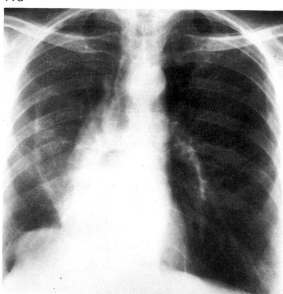

778 The anomalous vein is seen as a 'scimitar-like' shadow adjacent to heart border. Hypoplasia of the right lung is also present.

779

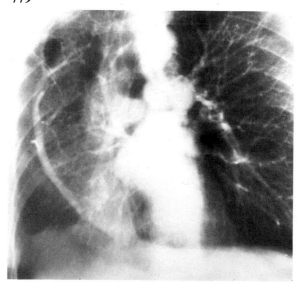

779 Angiogram shows drainage into the inferior vena cava. A significant left-to-right shunt may occur.

Foreign body in bronchus

A wide variety of foreign bodies may be inhaled. The airways are normally protected by the 'cough reflex', so most large foreign bodies are aspirated into the lungs of patients with reduced levels of consciousness.

780

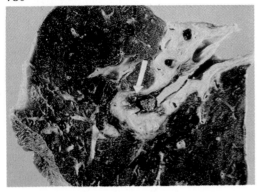

780   Hazelnut in bronchus of an alcoholic.

781

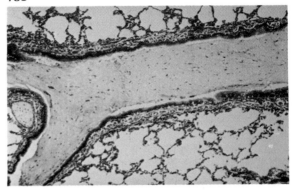

781   Brain tissue aspirated into bronchus of a child who sustained a fractured skull in a road traffic accident.

782

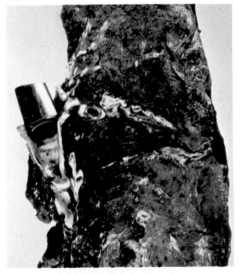

782   Pipe stem lying in major bronchus of a motor cyclist asphyxiated after inhaling fragments of pipe stem.

783

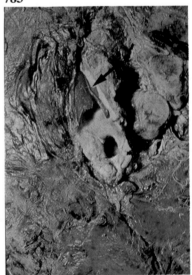

783   Red plastic cap inhaled into the bronchus of an epileptic.

Intrathoracic thyroid

Most examples of intrathoracic thyroids are caused by extensions of simple colloid goitres in the neck.

Insidious compression of the oesophagus may cause dysphagia; and of the trachea, dyspnoea and stridor. The great veins may also be compressed leading to superior vena-caval obstruction.

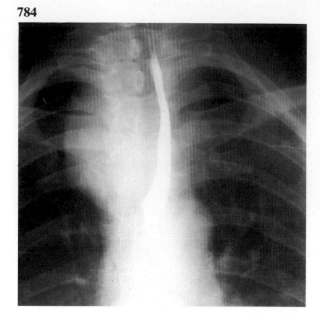

784   Barium swallow of oesophagus. The intrathoracic thyroid has displaced the oesophagus to the left.

Sequestration

Sequestration is a congenital abnormality of a portion of the lung, usually the lower lobe, which becomes isolated during development, so that the bronchi do not connect with the bronchial tree. Frequently the blood supply is abnormal; arising directly from the aorta.

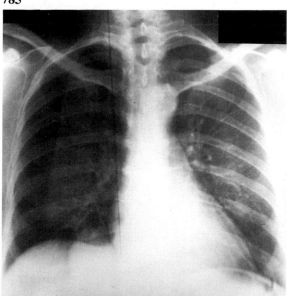

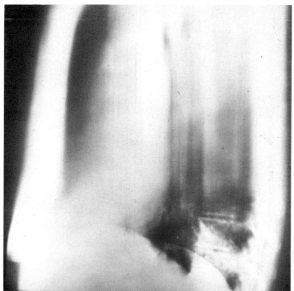

785 and 786   Sequestration of the posterior basal segment of the right lower lobe.

Thymoma

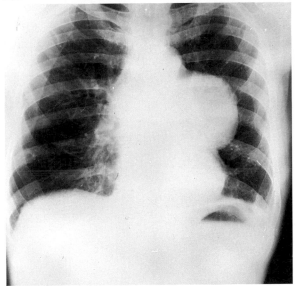

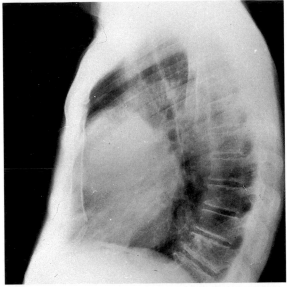

787 and 788 Xray of a large anterior mediastinal mass. A variety of cysts and tumours may occur in the mediastinum; especially lymphomas, metastatic carcinoma, teratomas and malignancies arising in the thyroid and thymus.

Surgery disclosed a solid tumour composed of reticular cells and lymphocytes (**789**); appearances typical of a thymoma. These tumours may be locally invasive and require postoperative radiotherapy.

Thymic tumours are found in up to 40 per cent of patients with myasthenia gravis (**790** and **791**) and may also be associated with hypogammaglobulinaemia, B-cell lymphopenia, systemic lupus erythematosus and polymyositis.

789 Thymoma. A solid tumour composed of reticular cells and lymphocytes.

789

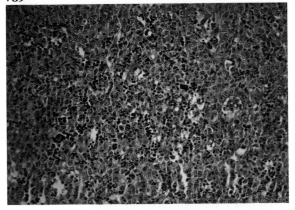

790

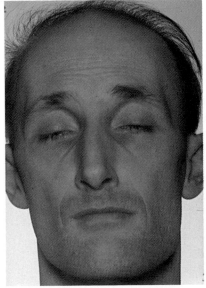

790 Myasthenia gravis. This is commonly associated with thymic tumours. Note the drooping eyelids and mouth.

791 Tensilon test for myasthenia gravis. The prompt relief of weakness supports the diagnosis. This patient was cured by thymectomy.

791

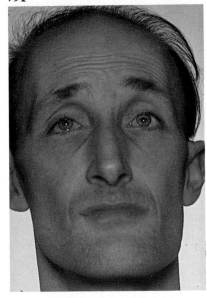

Pulmonary atresia

792

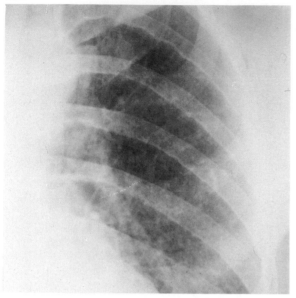

793

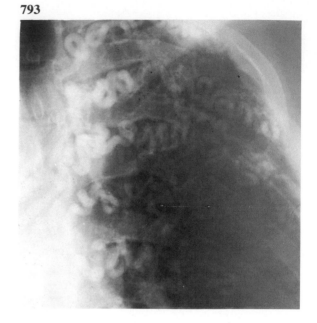

792 and 793 Pulmonary atresia. The PA film shows notching of the ribs. The aortic angiogram shows tortuous and dilated intercostal arteries. Rib notching can also occur in coarctation of the aorta.

Melkersson–Rosenthal syndrome

794 The Melkersson–Rosenthal syndrome (MRS). There is circumscribed oedema of the lips, periorbital tissues, forehead, gums, tongue, palate, throat, larynx and other cervicofacial tissues. The histology of this oedematous tissue is a granulomatous reaction so the disorder is sometimes mislabelled as sarcoidosis. It has also been labelled cheilitis granulomatosa. The tongue may exhibit macroglossia or a cobbled appearance (glossitis granulomatosa) or is fissured (lingua plicata). The salivary gland on the side of the oedema may have poor function whereas there is hypersalivation on the other side. Facial palsy as well as salivary and cervical gland involvement serve to heighten the similarity to sarcoidosis although they are quite unrelated. Additional features of MRS are bronchial asthma, transient fever and slightly elevated ESR.

The granuloma formation suggests an antigen-antibody reaction. There is also evidence of the presence of IgE-forming plasma cells and raised serum IgE.

794

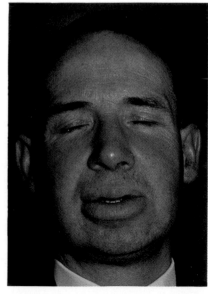

Index

The numbers in **bold** refer to figure numbers showing the relevant condition; the figures in medium type indicate page numbers where the condition is mentioned.